BUYING AN E-BIKE FOR SENIORS

Your passport to fun, freedom, and fitness at any age

By Scott Bourne

TABLE OF CONTENTS

Preface:
Rediscovering the Joy of Cycling

I remember the first time I rode a bicycle. The wind in my face, the whirring of the wheels, the incredible sense of freedom – it was pure magic. For many of us, as we get older, we might think those days are gone. Aches, pains, challenging hills, or simply the fear of not being able to keep up can put our beloved bikes in the garage to gather dust.

But what if I told you that you could recapture that magic? What if you could flatten those hills, cruise for miles with ease, and feel that same sense of exhilaration again, regardless of your age or current fitness level?

Welcome to the world of e-biking! (electric bikes)

As a 70-year-old cycling enthusiast myself, discovering e-bikes was a revelation. It wasn't about cheating; it was about enabling. It was about making cycling accessible, enjoyable, and sustainable again. It allowed me to keep riding, explore further, tackle those daunting Las Cruces mesas, and, most importantly, have a lot of fun doing it.

I wrote this book, Buying an E-bike for Seniors, because I want to share that discovery with you. Navigating the e-bike market can seem overwhelming at first. There are so many types, features, and technical terms. My goal is to demystify the process, cut through the jargon, and guide you step-by-step towards finding the perfect e-bike that fits your needs, your budget, and your dreams.

This book is your passport. It's your guide to understanding, choosing, and safely enjoying an e-bike. It's your invitation to rediscover fun, reclaim your freedom, and boost your fitness at any age.

Remember, it's never too late to roll

Scott Bourne Las Cruces, New Mexico, May 2025

Legal disclaimer and terms of use for "Buying an E-bike for Seniors"

Please read this disclaimer carefully before using this book.

Waiver and Release of Liability

In consideration for being permitted to use the information in this book, you, for yourself and for your heirs, next of kin, executors, administrators, legal representatives, assignees, and successors in interest (collectively "Releasors"), hereby WAIVE, RELEASE, DISCHARGE, HOLD HARMLESS, AND PROMISE NOT TO SUE the author, publisher, their respective agents, employees, officers, directors, contractors, and affiliates (collectively "Releasees") from any and all claims, demands, damages, losses, liabilities, actions, causes of action, suits, debts, sums of money, accounts, reckonings, bonds, bills, specialties, covenants, contracts, controversies, agreements, promises, variances, trespasses, judgments, executions, and expenses (including attorneys' fees and costs), of any nature whatsoever, in law or equity, whether known or unknown, suspected or unsuspected, which you ever had, now have, or hereafter can, shall, or may have for, upon, or by reason of any matter, cause, or thing whatsoever arising out of or relating in any way to your use of this book, your purchase or use of an e-bike, or your participation in cycling activities, including, but not limited to, any claims for personal injury, property damage, or wrongful death, whether caused by the negligence of the Releasees or otherwise.

Rider responsibility and safety precautions

It is your sole responsibility to ensure your own safety and the safety of others while cycling. The author and publisher strongly advise and insist that:

Always wear appropriate safety gear: You should always wear a properly fitted and certified bicycle helmet that meets current safety standards (e.g., CPSC, Snell, ASTM). The use of additional protective gear, such as gloves, eye protection, and appropriate footwear, is also highly recommended.

Read manufacturer's instructions: Before operating any e-bike, you must thoroughly read, understand, and follow all instructions, warnings, and safety information provided in the e-bike manufacturer's owner's manual and any other accompanying documentation.

Proper bike setup and maintenance: Ensure your e-bike is properly assembled, fitted to you, and regularly maintained according to the manufacturer's recommendations. This includes checking brakes, tire pressure, battery connections, and all other critical components before each ride. If you are unsure about any aspect of setup or maintenance, consult a qualified bicycle mechanic.

Obey all laws: Familiarize yourself with and obey all applicable local, state, and federal traffic laws, regulations, and ordinances pertaining to the operation of bicycles and e-bikes in your area.

Ride within your abilities: Assess your own physical condition, skill level, and the riding environment before and during each ride. Do not attempt maneuvers or ride in conditions that are beyond your capabilities.

Seek professional advice: The information in this book is not a substitute for professional advice. Consult with your physician before starting any new exercise program, including cycling. If you have any concerns about your ability to safely operate an e-bike, consult with a qualified cycling instructor or e-bike professional.

Not professional advice

The contents of this book are for informational purposes only and do not constitute professional mechanical, medical, legal, or financial advice. You should consult with a qualified professional for any such advice.

Limitation of liability

To the maximum extent permitted by applicable law, in no event shall the author or publisher be liable for any direct, indirect, punitive, incidental, special, or consequential damages, or any damages whatsoever, including, without limitation, damages for loss of use, data, or profits, arising out of or in any way connected with the use or performance of this book, with the delay or inability to use this book, or for any information, products, services, or related graphics obtained through this book, or otherwise arising out of the use of this book, whether based on contract, tort, negligence, strict liability, or otherwise, even if the author or publisher has been advised of the possibility of damages. Because some states/jurisdictions do not allow the exclusion or limitation of liability for consequential or incidental damages, the above limitation may not apply to you. If you are dissatisfied with any portion of this book, or with any of these terms of use, your sole and exclusive remedy is to discontinue using this book.

Indemnification

You agree to indemnify, defend, and hold harmless the author, publisher, and their respective officers, directors, employees, agents, licensors, suppliers, and any third-party information providers to the book from and against all losses, expenses, damages, and costs, including reasonable attorneys' fees, resulting from any violation of this disclaimer by you or any activity related to your use of the book (including negligent or wrongful conduct).

Governing Law and Jurisdiction

This disclaimer and any dispute or claim arising out of or in connection with it or its subject matter or formation (including non-contractual disputes or claims) shall be governed by and construed in accordance with the laws of the State of New Mexico, United States of America, without regard to its conflict of law provisions.

You agree that any legal action or proceeding between the author/publisher and you for any purpose concerning this disclaimer or the parties' obligations hereunder shall be brought exclusively in a federal or state court of competent jurisdiction sitting in the State of New Mexico.

Severability

If any provision of this disclaimer is found to be unlawful, void, or for any reason unenforceable, then that provision shall be deemed severable from this disclaimer and shall not affect the validity and enforceability of any remaining provisions.

Entire agreement

This disclaimer constitutes the entire agreement between you and the author/publisher with respect to your use of this book and supersedes all prior or contemporaneous communications and proposals, whether electronic, oral, or written, between you and the author/publisher with respect to this Book.

Acknowledgement

By purchasing, accessing, or using this book, you acknowledge that you have read this disclaimer, understand its terms, and agree to be bound by them. If you do not agree to these terms, do not use this book.

This disclaimer is subject to change without notice.

Last updated: August, 2025

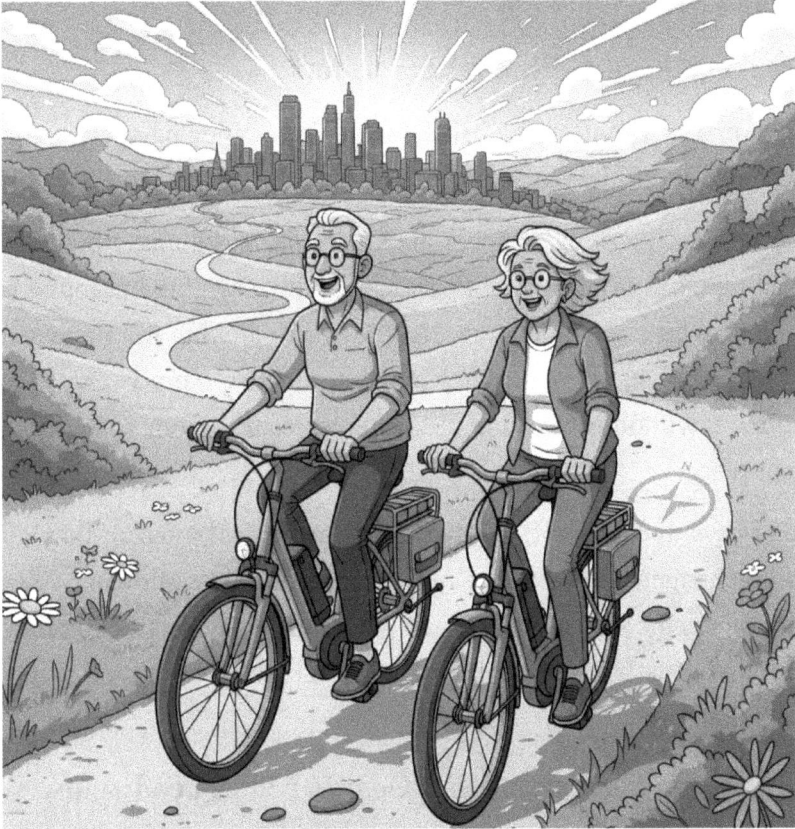

CHAPTER 1:
WHY AN E-BIKE NOW?

The benefits of e-bikes for 55+ riders

Welcome to Buying an E-Bike for Seniors: Your passport to fun, freedom, and fitness at any age

If you're reading this, chances are you're curious about e-bikes and what they can offer. Perhaps you used to love cycling but found it's become a bit too challenging. Maybe you're looking for a new way to stay active, explore your community, or simply enjoy the outdoors without overdoing it. Whatever your reason, you're in the right place!

For riders aged 55 and older, e-bikes aren't just a trend; they're a game-changer. They open a world of possibilities, allowing you to experience the joy of cycling in a whole new way. Let's explore the many reasons why an e-bike might be the perfect addition to your life right now.

1.1. Extend your riding life: Conquer hills, headwinds, and fatigue

Remember those long rides you used to love? Or perhaps you've always wanted to cycle more but found hills daunting, or strong winds made even short trips exhausting? This is where an e-bike truly shines.

An e-bike provides an electric "assist" that works with your pedaling. It's not a motorcycle. You still pedal, but the motor provides a gentle (or not-so-gentle, depending on your setting) push when you need it most. This means:

- Hills become manageable: That intimidating incline where you used to walk your bike? With an e-bike, you can often pedal right up it with a smile.
- Headwinds are no match: Battling a strong headwind can be incredibly tiring. The e-bike's motor helps you push through, keeping your momentum and energy up.
- Fatigue is reduced: You can ride longer distances or for more time without feeling completely worn out. This allows you to truly enjoy the scenery and the experience, rather than focusing on how tired your legs are.
- Keeping up is easy: If you ride with friends or family who are younger or fitter, an e-bike ensures you can keep pace effortlessly, making group rides more enjoyable for everyone.

Think of it as having a very friendly tailwind always at your back, ready to help when you need it.

1.2. Boost your health and fitness

Low-impact exercise, cardiovascular benefits, improved balance

One of the biggest misconceptions about e-bikes is that they do all the work for you. This couldn't be further from the truth! An e-bike is a fantastic tool for improving and maintaining your health and fitness, especially as we age.

You still pedal! The "assist" means you choose how much effort you put in. You can opt for minimal assistance for a good workout, or more assistance when you're feeling less energetic or tackling a tough section of road or trail. You're always in control of your workout level. This is even more true when you use what's known as a "torque sensor" to aid in your ride. More on that later.

Low-impact exercise. Cycling is inherently gentle on your joints, making it ideal for those with knee, hip, or back concerns. The e-bike's assist further reduces strain, allowing you to exercise without pain. This was key for me personally because I have very severe joint problems. If I didn't have my e-bike, I'd get no exercise.

Cardiovascular health. Regular cycling, even with assistance, elevates your heart rate, strengthening your heart and lungs. It's a great way to improve circulation and overall cardiovascular fitness.

Improved balance and coordination. Riding a bike naturally helps with balance. As you ride more frequently and confidently on an e-bike, you'll find your balance and coordination improving, which can have positive effects on your daily life.

(Another personal note here – I had a TBI more than a decade ago and it still slightly impacts my balance. Riding a three-wheeled trike – at first – led to me getting strong enough to add a two-wheeler to my garage. In other words, it did help with my balance.)

Mental well-being. Spending time outdoors, getting fresh air, and engaging in physical activity are proven mood boosters. E-biking can reduce stress, improve sleep, and provide a wonderful sense of accomplishment.

An e-bike empowers you to get the exercise you need and want, at a pace that's comfortable and sustainable for you. Once you start riding, this all gets magnified many times over.

1.3. Rediscover joy and freedom

Explore more, keep up, commute with ease

Remember the feeling of freedom you had on a bike as a child? An e-bike can bring that feeling right back!

Explore further. With the added power, you're no longer limited by distance or terrain. Discover new parks, trails, or neighborhoods that were previously out of reach. Take longer, more adventurous rides without worrying about the return journey.

Stay connected. Keep up with grandkids on their bikes, join friends for longer cycling excursions, or simply enjoy a leisurely ride with your partner. An e-bike ensures that you are part of the action.

Effortless commutes and errands. Need to pick up groceries? Want to visit a friend across town? An e-bike can make these short trips enjoyable and sweat-free, often faster than driving in traffic and easier than finding parking. Many e-bikes can be fitted with baskets or panniers (think saddle bags) to carry your essentials.

Pure enjoyment. The sheer pleasure of gliding along, feeling the breeze, and experiencing the world from a bicycle seat is amplified when you know you have the power to tackle any challenge the road throws at you.

An e-bike transforms cycling from a strenuous activity into a joyful, liberating experience.

1.4. Accessibility

Ideal for joint issues, limited stamina, or recovering from injuries

For many seniors, physical limitations can make traditional cycling difficult or impossible. E-bikes offer a wonderful solution, making cycling accessible to a wider range of individuals.

In my case, being overweight, 70 and having both joint and heart issues, on paper it looked like I was done. But the e-bike took me off that page and put me into a place where I felt like my old self again. It's one of the reasons I felt compelled to write this book. I wanted to share that information with anyone who would benefit from it.

Gentle on joints. As mentioned, cycling is low impact. The electric assist means less strain on your knees, hips, and ankles, allowing you to exercise without aggravating existing conditions.

Manages stamina. If your stamina isn't what it used to be, an e-bike allows you to regulate your effort. You can use more assist on days you're feeling less energetic or when you're just starting to ride, gradually building your endurance over time.

Recovery and rehabilitation: For those recovering from injuries or surgeries, an e-bike can be a fantastic tool for gentle rehabilitation, helping to rebuild strength and mobility without excessive stress. Always consult your doctor or physical therapist before starting any new exercise regimen.

Confidence builder: The added stability and power can significantly boost your confidence on two wheels, especially if you haven't ridden in a while or feel unsteady on a traditional bike. Many e-bikes also feature "step-through" frames, which make mounting and dismounting much easier and safer.

An e-bike isn't just a bike. It's an enabler, helping you overcome physical barriers and get back to enjoying life on two wheels.

1.5. Environmental perks – financial perks: A green alternative, saving on fuel

Beyond personal health benefits and enjoyment, choosing an e-bike also offers advantages for your wallet and the planet. If you live in an urban environment, it becomes much easier to see these benefits than if you live outside such an environment. But the potential is always there.

Reduce your carbon footprint. Opting for an e-bike instead of a car for short trips significantly reduces your emissions, contributing to cleaner air and a healthier environment. It's a small change that makes a big difference.

Save on fuel costs. Imagine how much you could save on gasoline if you used your e-bike for errands, commutes, or social visits instead of your car. These savings can add up quickly.

Lower maintenance than a car. While an e-bike requires some maintenance (which we'll cover later), it's generally far less expensive to maintain than a car.

Parking made easy (and free). Finding and paying for parking can be a hassle. With an e-bike, you can often park right where you need to be, for free.

An e-bike is an investment in your health, happiness, and a more sustainable lifestyle.

As you can see, the reasons to consider an e-bike are compelling, especially for riders aged 55 and over. It's about regaining freedom, boosting your well-being, and rediscovering the sheer joy of cycling. In the next chapter, I'll dive deeper into what an e-bike is, breaking down its key components in simple terms. Get ready to pedal!

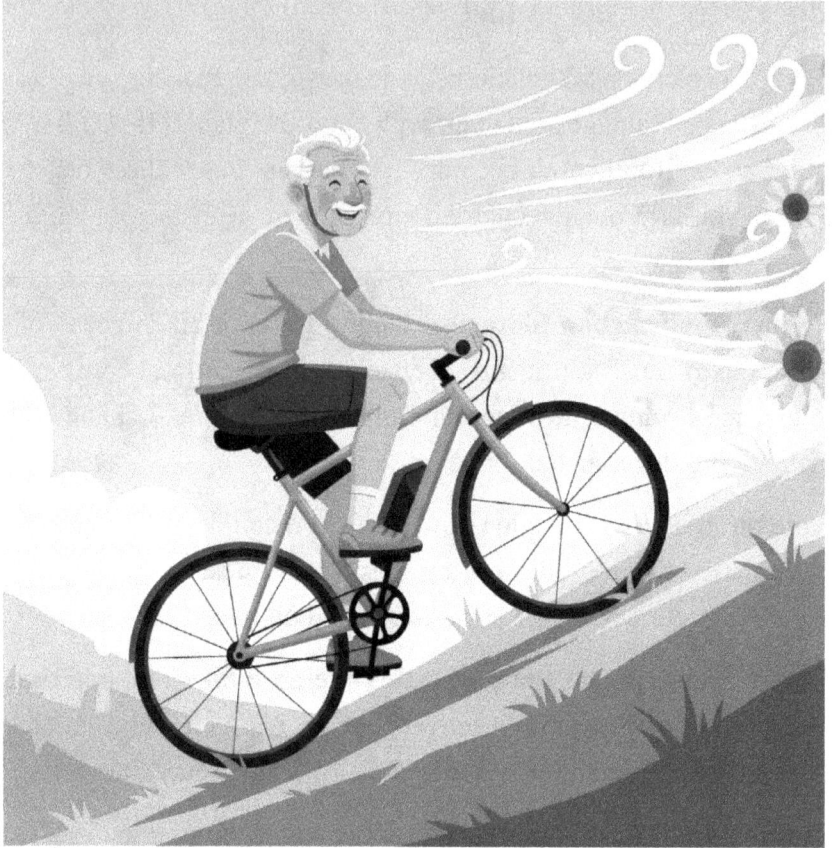

CHAPTER 2:
WHAT EXACTLY IS AN E-BIKE?

Unpacking the basics in the previous chapter, I talked about all the wonderful reasons why an e-bike might be perfect for you. Now, let's get down to the nuts and bolts. You might be wondering, "What is an e-bike, really? How does it work?"

Don't worry, I'm not going to dive into complex engineering. My goal here is to give you a clear, simple understanding of the main parts of an e-bike and how they work together to give you that amazing "pedal power reimagined" experience. Think of it as getting to know your new best friend before you go on adventures together!

2.1. The core concept: A bicycle with an electric motor to assist pedaling

At its heart, an e-bike is still a bicycle. It has pedals, wheels, tires, handlebars, and brakes – all the familiar parts you'd expect. The key difference, and what makes it "electric," is the addition of a few special components:

- An electric motor — This is the "engine" that provides the extra push.
- A battery — This powers the motor.
- A controller — This is the "brain" that manages how the motor and battery work together.
- Sensors — These tell the controller when and how much assistance to provide.

When you pedal, these components work in harmony to give you an extra boost. It's like having a very strong, invisible helper pushing you along, making hills feel flatter and distances shorter. You're still doing the pedaling, but with less effort, allowing you to go further, faster, and with more joy.

2.2. Key components explained

Your e-bike's essential parts: Let's look a little closer at these special components

The motor. The motor is where the power comes from to provide electric assistance. There are two main places you'll find the motor on an e-bike.

Hub Motors. These motors are built directly into the center (the "hub") of one of the wheels, usually the rear wheel.

Think of it like it's a tiny, powerful engine right inside your wheel.

Pros for seniors. Often more affordable, simpler design, and can provide a direct push feeling. If your chain breaks, you can still get some motor assist (if it has a throttle, which I'll discuss below).

Con. Can make the wheel feel heavier, and it's not always as smooth or efficient on very steep hills compared to mid-drive motors.

Mid-drive motors. These motors are in the middle of the bike, where the pedals (the "crank set") are. Think of it like an engine that works directly with your gears, amplifying each time you pedal.

Pros for seniors. Very efficient, especially on hills, as they use the bike's gears. This often provides a more natural, balanced riding feel. They can also be quieter.

Cons. Generally more expensive, and if your chain breaks, you lose all motor assist.

Which is better? For most senior riders, either can be excellent. Mid-drive motors often offer a more refined and powerful experience for hill climbing, while hub motors are a great, budget-friendly option for flatter terrain or casual rides. Don't let this decision overwhelm you. focus on how the bike feels when you test ride it.

Battery. The battery is your e-bike's fuel tank. It stores the electricity to power the motor. It's usually a sleek, rectangular pack often integrated into the bike's frame or mounted on a rack.

Capacity (watt-hours or Wh). This tells you how much energy the battery can hold, similar to how many gallons a car's fuel tank holds. A higher watt-hour number generally means a longer range.

Range. This is how far you can travel on a single charge. It varies greatly depending on the battery's capacity, how much assist you use, the terrain, your weight, and even the temperature. Most e-bikes offer ranges from 20 to 80 miles or more.

Cautionary Tip. Many e-bike manufacturers list the potential distance of a full battery charge based on a best-case scenario, i.e., a person weighing 150 pounds on a completely flat surface riding on a windless day and using a minimum amount of pedal assist. My personal experience indicates that I can expect about half the maximum advertised distance on any ride, and I act accordingly. You should start out as if your e-bike's battery will not perform as well as advertised. Then decide how far you want to go. On another note, many e-bikes can be fitted with a second or auxiliary battery that extends range.

Charging. E-bike batteries are rechargeable, just like your phone or laptop. They come with a special charger that plugs into a standard wall outlet. Charging times may vary but they typically take anywhere from two to eight hours. Many batteries can be removed from the bike for easier charging indoors.

Important tip: Always keep your battery charged, especially if you plan a longer ride. Think of it like topping up your car's gas tank before a road trip.

The controller and display: your command center. The controller is the "brain" of the e-bike. It's a small computer that manages the flow of power from the battery to the motor based on your input. You don't usually see the controller itself, but you interact with its output through the display.

The display is typically a small screen mounted on your handlebars. It shows you important information like:

Speed — How fast you're going.

Battery Level — How much charge you have left.

Assist Level — Which level of motor assistance you're currently using (e.g., Eco, Tour, Sport, Turbo).

Distance — How far you've ridden.

You'll usually have simple buttons near the display to turn the bike on/off, change assist levels, and cycle through information. Look for a display that's easy to read in different lighting conditions and buttons that are large and simple to operate while riding.

Sensors. Here's how your e-bike knows when to help. E-bikes use sensors to detect when you pedal and how much assistance to provide. There are two main types:

Cadence sensors. These are the most common and often found on more affordable e-bikes. They detect if you are pedaling. Once you start pedaling, the motor kicks in and helps.

Think of it like an on/off switch for the motor. If your feet are moving the pedals, you get power.

Pros for seniors. Simple, predictable assistance.

Cons: Can feel a little less natural, as the power might come on with a slight delay or continue for a moment after you stop pedaling.

Torque Sensors These are more sophisticated and usually found on higher-end e-bikes. They detect how hard you are pedaling. The harder you pedal, the more power the motor provides.

Think of it like an intelligent assistant that matches your effort.

Pros for seniors. Provides a very smooth, natural, and intuitive riding experience, making it feel more like you're just a super-strong cyclist.

Cons. Generally more expensive.

Which is better? Torque sensors offer a more seamless and natural feel, which many riders prefer. However, cadence sensors are perfectly functional and often found on excellent, more budget-friendly e-bikes. Again, test riding will help you decide which feel you prefer.

I started out with a cadence sensor, and I think it made the learning process easier. I now own a bike that offers both a cadence and a torque sensor. I occasionally use one or the other depending on how much of a workout I want to get.

2.3. Types of pedal assist vs. throttle

This is an important distinction when considering how you want your e-bike to deliver power.

Pedal Assist System (PAS). This is the most common type of e-bike operation. The motor only provides power when you are pedaling. You choose an assist level (e.g., "Eco" for light help, "Turbo" for maximum boost), and the motor adds power as you pedal. If you stop pedaling, the motor stops assisting.

Think of it like a constant boost that works with your leg power.

Pros for seniors. Encourages pedaling, extends battery life, and often feels more like a traditional bike ride. It's the most common and widely accepted type of e-bike.

Throttle. Some e-bikes also include a throttle, which can be a twist grip (like a motorcycle) or a thumb lever. With a throttle, you can engage the motor and get power without pedaling at all.

Think of it like a small scooter that you can also pedal.

Pros for seniors. Can be very helpful for getting started from a stop, especially on an incline, or for taking a quick break from pedaling. I use my throttle to launch myself on every ride – it's just easier than having to jump on the pedal hard to get rolling. I also use my throttle when I must ride at very slow speeds – to execute tight turns for instance. This allows me to make sure I have forward motion (super important if you don't want to fall over), and it gives me confidence that I need to get through tricky situations.

Cons. Using the throttle exclusively can drain the battery faster and means you're getting less exercise. Not all e-bike classes (see next section) allow throttles.

Many e-bikes offer both PAS and a throttle, giving you the best of both worlds.

2.4. E-bike classes (Class 1, 2, 3): What they mean for speed and where you can ride

E-bikes in the United States (and increasingly elsewhere) are often categorized into three classes. These classes primarily define the maximum speed at which the motor will assist you and whether it has a throttle. This is important because different classes may be allowed on different types of paths or trails.

Class 1 e-bike

Motor assistance. Only when you pedal (pedal assist).

Maximum assisted speed. Up to 20 mph.

Where you can ride. Generally allowed wherever traditional bicycles are allowed, including most bike paths and trails.

Think of it as the most "bicycle-like" e-bike.

Class 2 e-bike

Motor assistance. Both when you pedal (Pedal Assist) AND with a throttle.

Maximum assisted speed. Up to 20 mph (throttle or pedal assist).

Where you can ride. Similar to Class 1, generally allowed wherever traditional bicycles are allowed.

Think of it as a bike that can give you a boost even if you're not pedaling.

Class 3 e-bike

Class 3 e-bikes have powerful motor assistance. It is available when you pedal (Pedal Assist).

Maximum assisted speed. Up to 28 mph.

Where you can ride. Often restricted on bike paths and multi-use trails. More commonly allowed on roads. Some states or cities may require riders to be 16 or older and wear a helmet.

Think of it as a faster, road-focused e-bike.

Which class is right for you? For most senior riders, Class 1 or Class 2 e-bikes are typically the best choice. If for no other reason than to deal with a plethora of growing legal action against e-bikes, the safe bet is to avoid Class 3.

Class 1 and 2 are widely accepted on most bike paths and trails, and a top speed of 20 mph is plenty fast for comfortable, safe, and enjoyable riding. Unless you specifically plan to ride primarily on roads and desire higher speeds, a Class 3 e-bike might be unnecessarily restricted for your needs. Always check local regulations in your area, as rules can vary.

All my e-bikes have been Class 2 and I've never been restricted as to where I can ride, and I have never felt like I didn't have enough speed or power.

That was a lot of information, but now you have a solid foundation for understanding what makes an e-bike tick. You know about the motor, battery, display, and how the power is delivered. Most importantly, you understand the different classes and what that means for your riding adventures.

In the next part, I'll shift my focus to helping you choose the right e-bike for your needs, looking at different styles and features that are particularly beneficial for senior riders. Get ready to start thinking about your perfect ride!

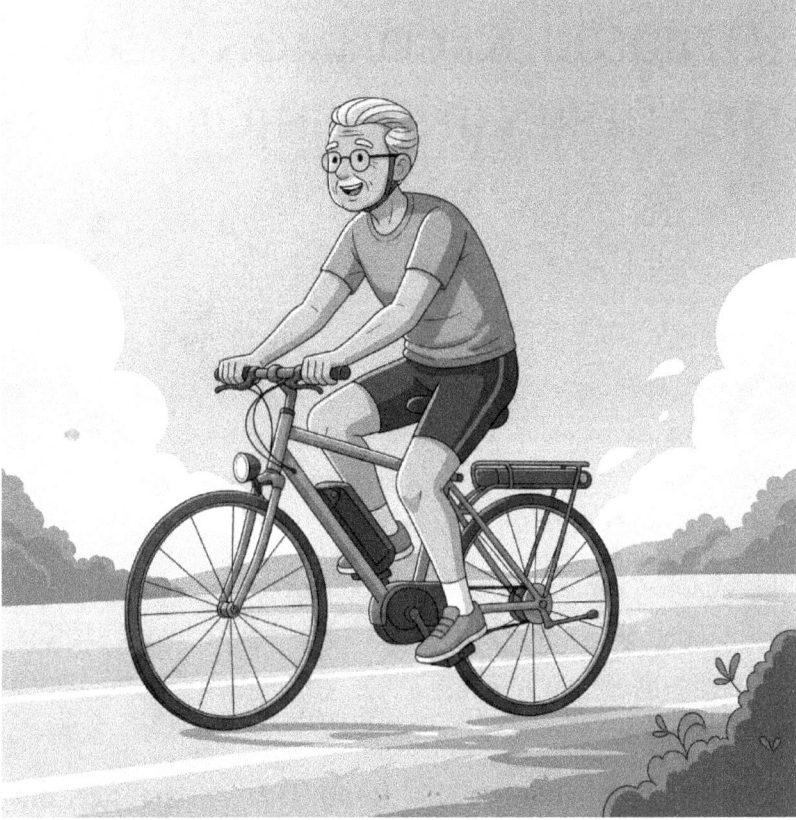

CHAPTER 3:
DEBUNKING COMMON MYTHS AND ADDRESSING SENIOR RIDERS' CONCERNS

It's completely natural to have questions, doubts, or even hear some common misconceptions when you're considering something new, especially a significant purchase like an e-bike. Many people, including those who haven't tried an e-bike themselves, might have opinions or outdated information.

In this chapter, I'm going to tackle some of the most frequent myths and concerns that senior riders often have about e-bikes. My goal is to provide you with accurate information and peace of mind so that you can make an informed decision with confidence.

3.1. Myth: "It's cheating!" – Reality: It's assistance, not replacement

This is perhaps the most common thing you'll hear about e-bikes, often from traditional cyclists. The idea is that if there's a motor, you're not really cycling, and therefore, it's "cheating."

The truth. An e-bike is designed to assist your pedaling, not replace it. You still must pedal, you still get exercise, and you're still in control of your effort level.

You're still active. Think of it like this: if you use an escalator to go up a flight of stairs, are you "cheating" at getting to the next floor? No, you're simply using a tool to make an activity more accessible and enjoyable. An e-bike is the same. You choose how much assistance you want. On "Eco" mode, you'll still be working quite hard, especially on hills. On "Turbo" mode, you'll feel like a superhero, but your legs are still turning the cranks!

More miles, more often. The "assist" means you can ride longer, go further, and tackle routes you might have avoided before. This often leads to more time exercising outdoors, not less. Many e-bike riders find they cycle more frequently and for longer durations than they ever did on a traditional bike.

It's about enjoyment, not competition. Unless you're a professional racer, cycling is about enjoyment, health, and freedom. An e-bike simply enhances these aspects, allowing you to get more out of your ride on your own terms.

Studies published by the International Journal of Behavioral Nutrition and Physical Activity, as well as studies by faculty at Brigham Young University found that e-biking is a legitimate form of exercise that can significantly contribute to physical activity levels and health, particularly by encouraging people to cycle more often and for longer distances than they might on a traditional bike. The "percentage" of exercise is hard to pin down with a single number due to the variables (assist level, terrain, rider effort, duration, frequency), but it's generally recognized as being within the moderate-to-vigorous intensity range.

So, next time someone says, "it's cheating," you can confidently tell them it's simply smart cycling, allowing you to extend your riding life and enjoy the outdoors more!

3.2. Concern: "They're too fast/dangerous!"

Reality: You control the speed, safety features are key

The idea of an electric motor might make you think of motorcycles or scooters, leading to concerns about excessive speed or lack of control.

The truth: You are always in control of your speed, and e-bikes come with excellent safety features. If the operator simply takes 20 minutes to read the manual and can operate a traditional bike, then there's nothing to be afraid of.

You set the pace. E-bikes don't just zoom off on their own. The motor only assists when you pedal (in pedal-assist mode) or when you engage the throttle (if your bike has one). You choose the assist level, which dictates how much power the motor adds. You can always ride at a comfortable, safe speed for the conditions and your skill level.

Speed limits are built in. As I discussed in Chapter 2, e-bikes are categorized into classes (Class 1, 2, and 3). Most e-bikes for recreational use (Class 1 and 2) will only assist you up to 20 mph. Beyond that speed, the motor stops assisting, and you're relying purely on your own leg power, just like a regular bike. This prevents unintended high speeds.

Superior braking systems. Many e-bikes, especially those designed for heavier loads or higher speeds, come equipped with powerful hydraulic disc brakes. These provide excellent stopping power, even in wet conditions, and require less hand strength to operate than traditional rim brakes. This is a significant safety advantage. These brakes are superior to those found on most traditional bicycles.

Weight adds stability. While e-bikes are heavier than traditional bikes, this added weight can contribute to a more stable ride, especially at lower speeds or when encountering small bumps.

With proper riding technique (which I'll cover in a later chapter) and the right safety gear, an e-bike is a very safe way to enjoy cycling.

3.3. Myth: "I won't get a workout!"

Reality: You still pedal, you choose the effort level

This myth goes hand-in-hand with the "cheating" accusation. People assume that because there's a motor, you're not expending any energy.

The truth: You absolutely will get a workout on an e-bike, and you have complete control over how intense that workout is.

It's still a bicycle: Every e-bike requires you to pedal to engage the motor (unless you're solely using a throttle, which is less common for exercise). Your legs are still doing work.

Adjustable effort: Think of the pedal assist levels (Eco, Tour, Sport, Turbo) as different gears for your workout.

Want a light, easy ride? Use a higher assist level.

Want a moderate workout? Choose a mid-level assist.

Want to challenge yourself but still conquer hills? Use a lower assist level and let your legs do more of the work.

I frequently alter my rides/workouts so that one day I operate my e-bike with the least amount of pedal assist available. The next day, I'll use more pedal assist and go for longer distances. It's all up to me. And likewise, if you buy an e-bike, it will all be up to you.

Consistency is key. The beauty of an e-bike is that it makes cycling more accessible and enjoyable. This means you're more likely to ride consistently, which is far better for your health than occasional, rides that are taxing and no fun. These kinds of rides leave you too exhausted to go out again. Regular, moderate exercise is incredibly beneficial for cardiovascular health, muscle strength, and overall well-being. And the exercise you like is the exercise you'll do.

Since I bought my latest e-bike, I've ridden an average of six miles each day, without a break for many months. The only exception was when I had a medical procedure, and the doctor told me to take it easy. (Trust me, that was more painful than the procedure. I miss my bike when I can't ride.)

Focus on the fun: Instead of dreading a tough hill, you can focus on the scenery, the fresh air, and the sheer joy of riding. You'll find yourself extending your rides, exploring new areas, and getting more exercise than you might have thought possible.

An e-bike helps you get the exercise you need, at the intensity you choose, making fitness a fun and sustainable part of your routine.

3.4. Concern: "They're too heavy/clunky!"

Reality: Modern designs are sleek and manageable.

Early e-bikes sometimes looked a bit bulky, with large batteries and visible motors. This might lead to concerns about them being difficult to handle or store.

The truth: E-bike design has come a long way! Modern e-bikes are much sleeker, and while they are heavier than traditional bikes, they are designed to be manageable.

Once again, you have a choice. If your budget allows, you can buy an e-bike that is surprisingly light. It just costs more to get one that meets that criteria.

Integrated design. Many newer e-bikes have batteries seamlessly integrated into the frame, making them look very similar to regular bicycles. Motors are also becoming smaller and more discreet.

Weight distribution. Manufacturers carefully design e-bikes to distribute the weight of the motor and battery optimally, ensuring a balanced and stable ride.

Step-through frames. As mentioned, many e-bikes feature "step-through" frames, which have a very low bar, making it incredibly easy to mount and dismount the bike without having to swing your leg high over the seat. This is a huge advantage for seniors, those with limited mobility, or anyone who simply prefers an easier way to get on and off.

On a personal note, without a step-through frame, I couldn't ride. My knees are shot and so is my right hip. I cannot bring my leg over the high bar of a traditional bike. The step-through gives me easy and safe access to the bike. I can mount and dismount with ease. If you're at all concerned about being able to handle an e-bike I highly recommend starting with a step-through model. There are many to choose from and at all price points.

The motor helps with the weight. While an e-bike might feel heavy when you're pushing it or lifting it, once you're riding and the motor assist kicks in, the weight largely disappears. The motor helps you accelerate and maintain speed, making the bike feel surprisingly nimble.

Folding options. If storage space is a concern, there are excellent folding e-bikes available that reduce to a surprisingly small size, perfect for apartments, RVs, or putting in the trunk of a car.

Don't judge an e-bike by its weight when stationary. The true test is how it feels when you're riding it, and you'll likely be pleasantly surprised.

3.5. Concern: "They're too expensive!"

Reality: Investment in health and enjoyment, long-term savings e-bikes can certainly have a higher upfront cost than a basic traditional bicycle, which can be a barrier for some.

The truth: While an initial investment is required, an e-bike can be seen as an investment in your health, happiness, and even offer long-term financial savings.

It's also worth noting that the average serious road biker will spend between $2,500 and $7,500 on their traditionally powered bikes. Very good e-bikes cost much less. It always depends on the level of quality and utility that you are looking for. My last e-bike purchase was the Velotric Nomad 2. With tax, shipping and a few accessories, I paid less than $2,200. My friends who ride road bikes all think that is a killer deal. Your perspective will guide your thinking here.

Not everything should or can be judged on price alone. There is a big difference between price and value. E-bikes have lots of hidden value. Here are a few examples...

Investment in well-being. Consider the cost in terms of improved health, increased mobility, reduced stress, and the sheer joy of rediscovering cycling. These benefits are invaluable.

Consider other hobbies/transportation. When compared to the cost of a gym membership, a new car, or even regular public transportation, an e-bike can be a very cost-effective alternative over time.

Fuel savings. If you use your e-bike for errands or short commutes instead of your car, the savings on gasoline alone can add up significantly over months and years.

Reduced wear and tear on your car. Using your e-bike for shorter trips means less mileage on your car, potentially extending its life and reducing maintenance costs.

Durability and longevity. E-bikes are built to last, with robust frames and components. With proper care, your e-bike can provide years of reliable enjoyment.

One more thing about e-bike pricing:

Just like cars, e-bikes come in a wide range of prices. You don't need the most expensive model to get a fantastic experience. There are many excellent, reliable e-bikes available at various price points to suit different budgets.

Think of an e-bike as a long-term investment in a more active, enjoyable, and independent lifestyle. If you spend $2,000 now and ride your bike for five years, your cost will average out to $400 a year – slightly more than a dollar a day – and in return you'll have the time of your life.

I hope this chapter has helped to ease any concerns you might have had about e-bikes. They are truly revolutionary for riders of any age but especially riders who are 55+. These bikes are designed with accessibility, safety, and enjoyment in mind. By understanding the facts, you can confidently move forward in your e-bike journey.

Coming up, I'll dive into the exciting process of choosing your first e-bike, exploring different styles and features that are particularly well-suited for riders aged 55 and over. Get ready to find your perfect match!

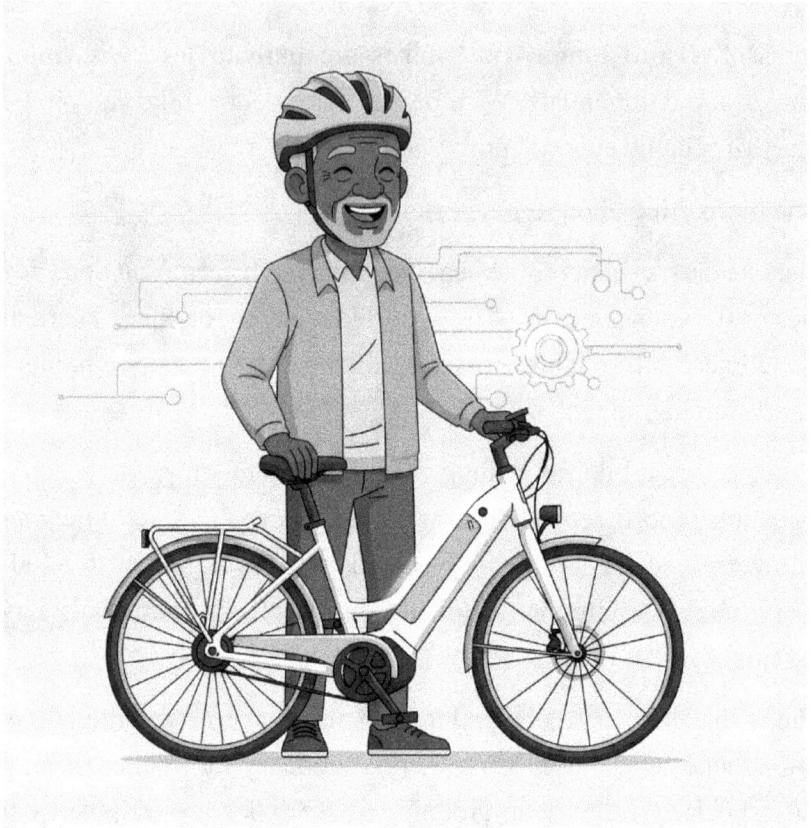

CHAPTER 4:
FINDING YOUR PERFECT FIT

The world of electric bicycles offers a diverse range of styles, each designed to cater to different needs and preferences. For seniors embarking on their e-bike journey, understanding these various types is crucial to finding a comfortable, safe, and enjoyable ride. This chapter will guide you through the most popular e-bike styles suitable for older adults, highlighting their key features and benefits, and helping you identify the perfect fit for your lifestyle.

4.1. Comfort and cruiser e-bikes

Upright riding, wide seats, easy step-through frames

Comfort and cruiser e-bikes are often the go-to choice for seniors, and for good reason. These bikes prioritize a relaxed and enjoyable riding experience above all else. Their design philosophy focuses on ease of use and maximum comfort, making them ideal for leisurely rides around the neighborhood, trips to the local shop, or scenic jaunts along paved paths.

Key features and benefits for seniors

Upright riding position. Perhaps the most significant advantage for many seniors is the upright riding posture. This design minimizes strain on your back, neck, and shoulders, allowing you to ride for longer periods without discomfort. It also provides excellent visibility of your surroundings.

Wide, padded seats. Comfort is the key benefit on these bikes, and this is reflected in their generous, well-padded saddles. These seats offer excellent support and cushioning, ensuring a pleasant ride even on longer excursions.

Easy step-through frames. A low or non-existent top bar makes mounting and dismounting these e-bikes effortless. This feature is particularly beneficial for seniors who may have concerns about balance or flexibility, significantly reducing the risk of falls when getting on or off the bike.

Swept-back handlebars. These handlebars allow your arms to remain in a natural, relaxed position, further contributing to a comfortable ride.

Wider tires. Cruiser e-bikes often feature wider tires that provide a smoother ride by absorbing bumps and imperfections in the road surface.

Simple controls. The focus is on ease of use, so these bikes typically have straightforward controls for adjusting the level of electric assistance.

Cruisers are ideal for seniors seeking a relaxed, comfortable, and easy-to-manage e-bike for leisurely rides on paved surfaces.

4.2. Hybrid and commuter e-bikes

Versatile for roads and light trails, good for daily use.

Hybrid and commuter e-bikes offer a versatile blend of features, making them a popular choice for seniors who plan to use their e-bike for a variety of purposes. These bikes strike a balance between the comfort of a cruiser and the efficiency of a road bike, making them suitable for both paved roads and light, well-maintained trails. They are excellent companions for daily errands, commuting, or longer recreational rides.

Key features and benefits for seniors

Balanced riding position. Hybrid e-bikes typically offer a more upright riding position than a road bike but are slightly more forward-leaning than a cruiser. This provides a good compromise between comfort and pedaling efficiency.

Versatile tires. These bikes usually come equipped with tires that are wide enough to handle a variety of surfaces but still offer good rolling resistance for efficient riding on pavement.

Multiple gearing options. Hybrid e-bikes often have a wider range of gears compared to cruisers, making it easier to tackle hills and varied terrain.

Mounting points for accessories. Commuter-focused hybrids often include mounting points for racks, fenders, and lights, making them practical for carrying groceries or riding in different weather conditions.

Responsive handling. They generally offer more agile handling than cruisers, which can be beneficial when navigating through urban environments or on winding paths.

Hybrid and commuter e-bikes are ideal for seniors looking for a versatile e-bike that can handle a mix of paved roads and light trails, suitable for both recreational rides and practical daily use.

4.3. Folding e-bikes

Portability for recreational vehicles (RVs), apartments, or multi-modal transport

For seniors with limited storage space or those who enjoy traveling and want to take their e-bike along wherever they go, folding e-bikes offer an ingenious solution. These bikes are designed to be compact and easily transportable, making them ideal companions for RV adventures, apartment living, or combining cycling with public transport. They also fit easily on most bike carriers and even on public transit like train, bus, and ferry systems.

Key features and benefits for seniors

Compact and portable. The primary advantage is their ability to fold down into a much smaller size, making them easy to store in closets, car trunks, or RV compartments.

Lightweight options. Many folding e-bikes are designed to be relatively lightweight, further enhancing their portability and making them easier to lift and carry.

Ease of transport. Their compact size allows for easy transport on buses, trains, or in the back of a car, opening new possibilities for exploration.

Suitable for shorter rides. While not always designed for long-distance touring, folding e-bikes are perfect for shorter commutes, errands, and exploring new destinations once you've arrived.

Step-through options. Many folding e-bike models also incorporate step-through frames, enhancing their accessibility for seniors.

Folding e-bikes are ideal for seniors who value portability, have limited storage space, or enjoy traveling and want to incorporate e-biking into their adventures.

4.4. Cargo e-bikes

For carrying groceries, grandkids, pets.

Cargo e-bikes are the workhorses of the e-bike world, designed to carry significantly more than just the rider. While they might not be the first choice for every senior, they can be an excellent option for those who want to replace car trips for grocery shopping, transport grandchildren, or simply carry a bit extra on their rides.

Key features

Extended frames. These bikes often have longer wheelbases and reinforced frames to accommodate cargo.

Integrated racks or baskets. Many come with built-in racks or large baskets for carrying goods.

Powerful motors. They are typically equipped with robust motors to handle the extra weight of cargo.

Considerations for seniors. Due to their size and weight, cargo e-bikes can be less easy to maneuver, but they offer other benefits.

For those with specific hauling needs, cargo e-bikes offer a practical and eco-friendly solution.

4.5. Mountain e-bikes

For adventurous off-roaders

For seniors with a spirit of adventure and a love for the great outdoors, electric mountain bikes (e-MTBs) open a world of off-road exploration. These bikes are specifically designed to tackle challenging trails, steep inclines, and uneven terrain.

Key features

Robust suspension. E-mountain bikes feature advanced suspension systems to absorb bumps and provide a smooth ride on rough trails.

Knobby tires. These tires offer excellent grip and traction on loose or uneven surfaces.

Powerful motors and brakes. They are equipped with powerful motors to assist on steep climbs and strong brakes for controlled descents.

Considerations for seniors. Mountain biking requires a certain level of fitness, balance, and skill.

While e-mountain bikes make off-road riding more accessible, it's essential for seniors to choose trails appropriate for their abilities and ride within their comfort zones.

One more thing...

Don't get too caught up in all these descriptions. They are descriptions of bicycles – not a description of you. If you own a mountain bike that doesn't necessarily mean you have to take on the persona of a mountain biker. Don't decide that you need to define yourself based on any of them. In other words, define the bikes – not yourself. For instance, I ride two different e-bikes. One is a three-wheeler with a cargo basket on the back – a trike. And I ride an e-mountain bike – also called a fat-tire bike.)

The trike is straight forward. I ride it casually and mainly used it to rehab myself when recovering from some medical problems. On the e-mountain bike, I have the handlebars raised and swept back, and I have installed a very wide (and heavily padded) seat. I generally treat this bike like a cross between a cargo bike and a cruiser.

You can customize any bike to your specific needs, so just look at this section of the book as a very brief introduction into e-bike types. Then look at what YOU want to do, what you want to accomplish, and what suits you best.

By carefully considering your needs, preferences, and intended use, you can confidently find the perfect match to embark on your e-bike journey.

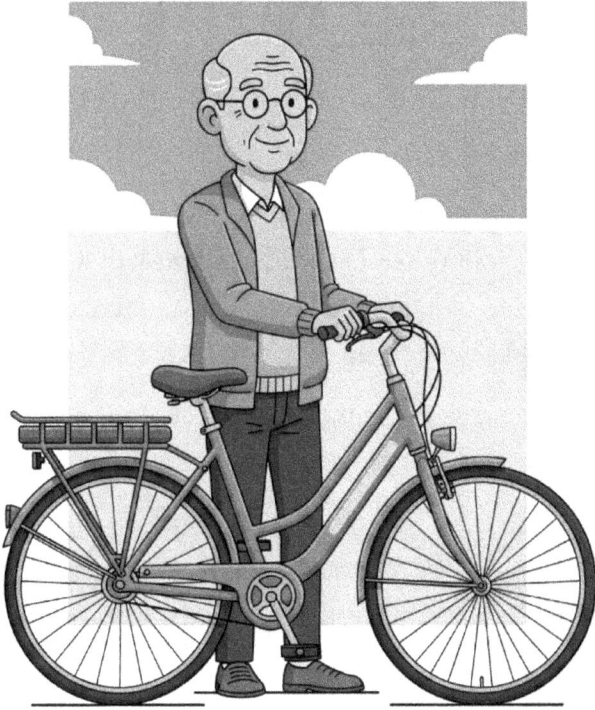

CHAPTER 5:
IDENTIFYING THE KEY FEATURES THAT MATTER

(I mean - What really matters)

Choosing your first e-bike involves more than just picking a style. It's about understanding the key features that will make your rides safe, comfortable, and enjoyable. With a myriad of technical specifications and a wide range of options, it can feel overwhelming.

This chapter will break down the essential components and features to consider, with a particular focus on what truly matters for senior riders.

By understanding these elements, you can make an informed decision and select an e-bike that perfectly suits your needs and preferences.

5.1. Frame design

The frame is the heart of your e-bike, influencing its handling, comfort, and ease of use. For seniors, certain frame design aspects are particularly crucial.

Step-through vs. step-over:

Spend a great deal of time thinking about this before you make a purchase decision!

One of the most significant considerations for many seniors is how easy it is to get on and off the e-bike. This is where the distinction between step-through and step-over frames becomes vital.

Step-through frames feature a very low or non-existent top tube, allowing you to easily "step through" the frame to mount and dismount. This design is highly recommended for seniors as it minimizes the need to lift your leg high, reducing the risk of losing balance or falling, especially when starting or stopping. Many comfort and cruiser e-bikes, as well as some hybrids and folding models, offer step-through designs.

Personal note – I never imagined I wouldn't be able to lift my leg over the top rail of a "men's" bicycle and hop on for a ride. Then osteoarthritis paid me a visit. It is the most common form of arthritis, affecting millions of people worldwide. It happens when the protective cartilage that cushions the ends of the bones wears down over time.

Although osteoarthritis can damage any joint, the condition most commonly affects joints in the hands, knees, hips, and spine. In my case it's mostly my knees.

Because of this, I can't step over the frame of an appropriately sized, men's bicycle. If it were not for the step-through style, I couldn't ride.

The good news is that staying active, maintaining a healthy weight, and receiving certain treatments might slow progression of the disease and help improve pain and joint function. In other words, riding my e-bike is making things better for me.

The most common form of bicycle (e-bike or not) is the step-over frame. These frames have a traditional diamond-shaped design with a higher top tube that you need to "step over" to mount. While often associated with a sportier look and potentially offering a slightly stiffer frame, they can be more challenging for seniors with limited flexibility or balance concerns. My highest recommendation is this.

If you are 55+ - even if you can this day step over the frame, buy a step-through frame e-bike. At some point (and probably sooner than you realize) you will need it. Most senior riders I've spoken with agree that this is the most practical and confidence-inspiring choice.

Next up: Consider what material is used to construct the frame.

The material of the frame impacts both the weight and durability of your e-bike. The two most common materials you'll encounter are:

Aluminum. This is the most popular choice for modern e-bike frames. It offers an excellent balance of strength, durability, and relatively low weight. Aluminum frames are generally more affordable than carbon fiber and lighter than steel.

Steel. Known for its exceptional durability and comfortable ride quality (as it tends to absorb some road vibrations), steel frames are often found on cruisers and some hybrid e-bikes. However, steel is heavier than aluminum, which can be a consideration when it comes to circumventing obstacles and transporting your e-bike.

My suggestion is that most seniors should strongly consider an aluminum frame. That choice provides a good blend of practicality and performance. If a very smooth ride is your top priority and weight isn't a major concern, a steel frame can also be a good option. I didn't mention carbon fiber much because frankly, I don't know of an e-bike with a carbon fiber frame and if there is one, you can bet it's incredibly expensive.

Adjustability

To ensure a comfortable and ergonomic riding position, look for an e-bike with good adjustability, particularly in the seat post and handlebars.

A quick-release seat post allows you to easily adjust the seat height without tools, making it simple to find the optimal leg extension for efficient and comfortable pedaling.

Adjustable handlebars, both in terms of height and reach (how far forward or backward they sit) allow you to fine-tune your riding posture. This is especially important for achieving an upright position that minimizes strain on your back and shoulders. I always look for this level of adjustability as a minimum standard.

5.2. Motor & Battery

The power behind your pedals

The motor and battery are what set an e-bike apart. Understanding their key characteristics will help you choose an e-bike that provides the right amount of assistance and range for your riding style.

Motor placement (hub vs. mid-drive and pros and cons for senior riders). E-bike motors are typically located in one of two places— the hub of one of the wheels (hub-drive) or near the pedals in the center of the bike (mid-drive).

Hub motors

These are often found on more affordable e-bikes and are generally simpler in design.

Pros: These are lower cost and can provide a "push" or "pull" feeling depending on whether it's in the rear or front hub, and they're often quieter.

Cons: Changing a flat tire can be more complex, weight distribution can be less balanced, and it may not feel as natural as mid-drive.

Mid-drive motors

These motors apply power directly to the crank set (where the pedals are).

Pros: These generally provide a more natural and intuitive riding feel and are often more efficient on hills as they leverage the bike's gears. Better weight distribution can offer improved handling.

Cons: These are typically more expensive and can put more strain on the chain and gears.

Recommendation for seniors

While both have merits, mid-drive motors often provide a more balanced and intuitive riding experience, which can be particularly beneficial for seniors. However, a good quality hub motor can still be a very suitable and more budget-friendly option. It's highly recommended to test ride both types to see which feels more comfortable and natural to you.

Battery capacity. (watt-hours and realistic range expectations). Battery capacity is measured in watt-hours (Wh). A higher Wh rating generally means a longer range. However, the actual range you get will depend on several factors:

Level of assistance. Using higher levels of assistance will drain the battery faster.

Terrain. Riding on hills will consume more battery power than riding on flat ground.

Rider weight and cargo. Heavier loads require more power.

Wind conditions. Riding into a headwind will increase battery usage.

Tire pressure. Properly inflated tires offer less resistance and improve range.

Realistic range expectations. While some manufacturers might claim very high ranges, it's important to have realistic expectations. For most seniors, a battery with a capacity of 400Wh to 500Wh will likely provide sufficient range for typical rides. It's always a good idea to inquire about the estimated "real-world" range based on different riding conditions.

Charging time and portability. Consider how long it takes to fully charge the battery and whether the battery is removable.

Charging Time

Most e-bike batteries take between three and six hours to fully charge. Faster charging can be convenient, but it's usually not a critical factor unless you plan on very long rides with quick turnarounds.

Portability

A removable battery allows you to bring it inside for charging, which is especially convenient if you store your e-bike in a garage or shed without easy access to an outlet. It also makes it easier to charge a spare battery if you choose to purchase one.

I suggest that you look for a removable battery for easier charging and consider a battery capacity that aligns with your anticipated riding distances.

5.3. Brakes

Reliable brakes are non-negotiable on any bicycle, and they are especially critical on d-bikes due to their potentially higher speeds and increased weight. Think of your brakes as your safety net on wheels.

Hydraulic disc brakes (highly recommended)

Hydraulic disc brakes are widely considered the gold standard for e-bikes. They offer superior stopping power. This is especially Important for e-bikes because they tend to be much heavier than non-e-bikes.

Hydraulics operate using hydraulic fluid, like the brakes in your car, and offer several key advantages:

Superior Stopping Power: They provide significantly more stopping power than other brake types, which is crucial for controlling the momentum of a heavier e-bike.

Excellent modulation. They allow for very precise control over your braking, letting you apply just the right amount of stopping force.

Consistent performance. They perform reliably in all weather conditions, including rain and mud.

Less hand effort required. They require less hand strength to operate, which can be a significant benefit for seniors.

Mechanical disc brakes vs. rim brakes

Mechanical disc brakes. These brakes use a cable to activate the brake calipers. They offer better performance than rim brakes, especially in wet conditions, but generally provide less power and modulation than hydraulic disc brakes. They are often found on more budget-friendly e-bikes.

Rim brakes. These brakes work by squeezing pads against the rim of the wheel. They are less common on modern e-bikes due to their reduced stopping power, especially in wet weather and with the added weight of an e-bike.

Recommendation: For the best in safety and performance, strongly prioritize e-bikes equipped with hydraulic disc brakes.

5.4. Gears and drivetrain

Gears play a crucial role in helping you maintain a comfortable pedaling cadence, especially when tackling hills or riding on varied terrain. The more gears your bike has, the easier it is to peddle.

You want to make sure you have enough gears for varied terrain unless you only do one kind of riding.

Most e-bikes come with a range of gears. While you might not need a huge number of gears (thanks to the electric assist), having enough options to comfortably handle inclines without straining yourself is important. For most seniors, a system with seven to nine gears is generally sufficient for a variety of riding conditions.

You'll need to decide what kind of shifting mechanism works best for you.

There are two main types of shifters.

Twist shifters. These work by twisting a section of the handlebar grip. They are often considered very intuitive and easy to use, especially for those who may have some hand dexterity issues.

Trigger shifters. These use small levers that you push with your thumb or forefinger to change gears. They can offer very precise shifting but may require a bit more practice for some users.

Recommendation: Twist shifters are often a good starting point for seniors due to their simplicity. However, it's worth trying both types to see which feels more comfortable and intuitive for your hands.

5.5. Suspension

A suspension system helps to absorb bumps and vibrations from the road or trail, leading to a more comfortable and controlled ride. Not all e-bikes have a suspension system. In fact, most lower-priced e-bikes do not. But for the ones that do, here's what you'll find.

Front suspension fork. This absorbs bumps and offers a smoother ride. A front suspension fork located on the front wheel is a common feature on many hybrids and some comfort e-bikes. It absolutely does help to soak up impacts from potholes, cracks, and uneven surfaces, reducing any jolts you feel through the handlebars and making your ride significantly smoother, especially on less-than-perfect roads.

How well this system works depends on the quality of the suspension and the weight of the rider. The heavier you are, the less reliably the front suspension will work to smooth out your ride.

If you weigh less than 250 pounds, there is a kind of "poor man's" suspension, and it's called a seat post suspension. It can be added to any bike. Some e-bikes like my Velotric Nomad II have a built-in seat post suspension. This provides an extra layer of cushioning directly under your seat, further enhancing comfort, particularly on longer rides or over bumpy terrain.

Rear shock

Some of the more expensive e-bikes may offer a rear shock. I have no experience with these systems, but my friends who have them swear by them. The problem is that you will have to add significantly to your budget to get one, so I'll leave this alone for now. But if you have questions about rear shocks on e-bikes, email me and I'll try to help.

My advice is that if you can afford it, get an e-bike with a front suspension fork. It is highly recommended for most seniors to improve comfort and control. You may want instead of, or in addition to that fork, a simple seat post suspension, which is (for most people) a valuable bonus feature that can further enhance your riding experience.

On my Velotric Nomad II, I have both a front fork suspension and a seat post suspension. The bike is the most comfortable to ride of any bike I've ever owned. I have about $2,700 in that bike, but you can buy it for $2,200 without all the accessories I have.

5.6. Tires

The tires on your e-bike play a crucial role in comfort, stability, and traction. They are your literal connection to the road and in my opinion, the most important part of the bike.

Not all tires (or wheels) are created equally. You need to think about tire size, width, tread, and tubed or tubeless.

Both of my e-bikes have 4"-wide tires. The wider tires generally offer more comfort and stability as they provide a larger contact patch with the ground and can be run at lower pressures, which helps to absorb bumps. You don't need to go that wide for comfort, but it helps. Look for tires that are a minimum of 2-inches wide for a good balance of comfort and efficiency.

For most seniors riding on paved surfaces or light trails, a tire with a smooth or semi-slick tread will provide good rolling efficiency and sufficient grip. If you plan on riding on more varied or unpaved surfaces, a tire with a more pronounced tread pattern might be beneficial.

I own a bike that is sold as a gravel or mountain bike, but I ride it almost exclusively on the street. I like having options and give up a little speed for a lot of safety and comfort. If speed is your deal, go for narrow tire widths.

Whatever tire you pick – know this. You WILL eventually get a flat tire. I like to say there are only two kinds of bicycle riders—those who have had a flat and those who are going to get a flat. Flat tires are a hassle for any cyclist.

Many e-bike tires now come with built-in puncture-resistant layers. This is a highly desirable feature as it can significantly reduce the likelihood of getting a flat, giving you more peace of mind on your rides. You can get tire inserts to help protect against flats. Flat-Out and Slime are two commercial products that can also help protect against flats. (I use Flat Out QuickStrike Tire Sealant Off-Road Formula (https://amzn.to/3SIwLmi) and went from two flats a week to no flats for the entire month. You can either learn how to add the sealant yourself or ask your bike mechanic to fill your tires with something like this. It will keep your bike on the road and out of the shop.

I also want to talk a bit about tread patterns. I suggest you opt for wider tires with a suitable tread pattern for your intended riding style and surface. I'd also prioritize tires with puncture resistance.

5.7. Display and controls:

Just like a car has a dashboard, your new e-bike will likely have a display and dashboard. The display and controls are your interface with the e-bike's electric system. They should be easy to see and use.

Look for a display that is bright and easy to see outdoors. Make sure it's readable and that it has a user-friendly layout. Look for an e-bike with a display that's easy to read at a glance.

Key features to consider

Large font size. Makes it easier to see important information like speed, battery level, and assistance level.

Clear and bright display. A backlit or high-contrast display is essential for good visibility in various lighting conditions.

Essential information. Ensure the display clearly shows your speed, battery level, and the current level of pedal assistance.

Ease of use (simple buttons, intuitive layout). The controls for adjusting the assistance level and turning the e-bike on and off should be intuitive and easy to operate without taking your hands too far from the handlebars.

5.8. Integrated lights and fenders

These features might seem like accessories, but for practical and safe e-biking, they are often essential for safety and or legal reasons.

Integrated lights are usually built-in front and rear lights that run off the e-bike's main battery and are a significant safety feature. They ensure you can see and be seen, both during the day and in low-light conditions. Some jurisdictions require lights on at night and a few require lights during the day.

Fenders (some call them mudguards) protect you from road spray and dirt, keeping you cleaner and more comfortable, especially when riding after rain or through puddles. They also can help protect the finish of your bike.

While not necessary, if you live somewhere that has a particularly rainy climate, or you ride in mud or dirt or on gravel, I think fenders are pretty much a must-have.

In any event, I always recommend that you consider e-bikes that come with integrated lights and fenders as standard equipment. This will save you the hassle and expense of adding them later and ensure they are properly integrated into your e-bike's design.

I cannot possibly mention all the nuances that go into picking a bike, but I've tried to list those things that I think are important, and I hope this list will help.

By carefully considering these key features, you'll be well-equipped to choose an e-bike that not only meets your needs but also enhances your riding experience, opening up a new world of active and enjoyable mobility.

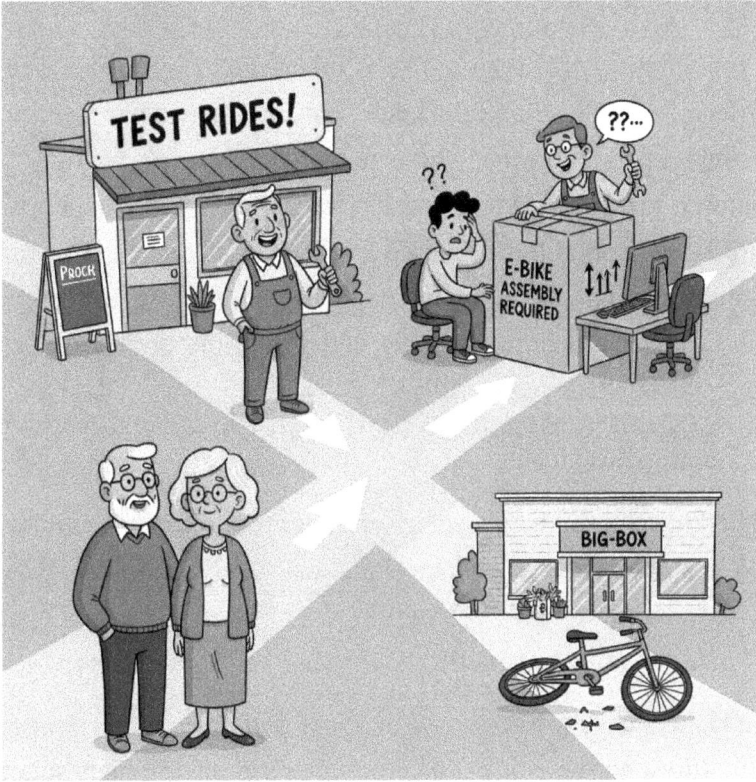

Chapter 6:
Where to Buy Your E-Bike

So, you've decided that an e-bike is the perfect way to embrace the joy of cycling with a helpful boost! That's wonderful news. The next exciting step is choosing where to purchase your new ride. This decision is just as important as selecting the right model, since it can significantly impact your overall experience, from initial setup to long-term enjoyment and maintenance. Next, we'll explore the most common places to buy an e-bike and weigh the pros and cons of each, especially for senior riders.

6.1. Local bike shops

(Highly recommended for seniors) For most seniors, I wholeheartedly recommend starting – and likely finishing – your e-bike search at a reputable local bike shop. These dedicated cycling hubs offer invaluable benefits that are hard to replicate elsewhere.

Even if the local shop charges a bit more than the online companies, you'll almost certainly still come out ahead given the local support.

The staff at a good local bike shop are passionate cyclists and e-bike experts. They can listen to your needs, understand your physical requirements (perhaps concerns about balance, flexibility, or strength), and guide you toward models that will be safe, comfortable, and enjoyable. They can answer your questions in person, demonstrate features, and explain the differences between various motor types, battery sizes, and frame styles.

After all that, the big benefit of buying local is getting an e-bike assembled. E-bikes, with their added motors and electronic components, are more complex than traditional bicycles. When you buy from a local bike shop, your e-bike will be professionally assembled and safety-checked by trained mechanics. This ensures everything from the brakes and gears to the electrical system is working correctly and safely from your very first ride, offering crucial peace of mind.

If you don't buy locally, you might just be fine. But what if there's a warranty claim? Who will take care of that? Will the manufacturer try to claim the bike wasn't properly assembled since you did it yourself and deny your claim? Who will do the labor if there is warranty work? All these questions evaporate if you buy locally.

Test rides

This is perhaps the most important reason to visit a local bike shop. How an e-bike looks on a screen or in a brochure can be very different from how it feels to ride. A local bike shop allows you to try out several different models. You can feel the weight, test the balance, see how easy it is to get on and off (consider step-through frames), experience how the motor engages, and check the comfort of the saddle and handlebars. You wouldn't buy a car without a test drive, and the same principle applies here.

I found out first-hand what a risk it is buying a bike sight unseen. One of my first e-bikes was bought online from a good company but I hadn't fitted the bike. When it arrived it was simply a horrible fit for me—too small and not what I wanted. I sold it but took a bath on it. The next time I wanted a bike I drove six hours to test it. Worth it!

As part of the test ride, a good local shop will spend time fitting you to the bike. Comfort and safety often come down to having an e-bike that fits your body properly. Bike shop staff can perform a professional fitting, adjusting the seat height and angle, handlebar position, and other elements to match your proportions and riding style. A proper fit prevents aches and pains, makes it easier to stay on the bike longer, improves control, and makes riding much safer and more enjoyable, especially on longer journeys.

If you do need service after the sale, the local shop is your best bet. Most e-bikes should be professionally checked and given a light tune-up after the first 100 miles. If you don't do this, some bike manufacturers won't honor the warranty. Beyond tune-ups, if you have a question about the battery or need some other repair, your bike shop is your go-to resource. Building a relationship with a local shop means you have trusted professionals nearby to handle maintenance, repairs, and warranty issues. They can also offer tips on local riding routes, safety gear, and accessories.

I'll say it again - While prices might sometimes be slightly higher than online, the value you receive in terms of expertise, assembly, test rides, fitting, and ongoing support often make the local shop the wisest and most rewarding investment for senior e-bike riders.

6.2. Online retailers

The internet offers a vast selection of e-bikes, often at competitive prices. While this can be tempting, it comes with considerations, especially for seniors.

Pros

You'll find brands and models online that might not be available in your local shops. You may find bikes in-stock online that aren't in-stock at your local dealer and there are potentially prices because online retailers often have lower overhead costs, which can sometimes translate into lower prices or frequent sales.

Cons

No matter what they promise, you will have to do SOME assembly of your e-bike. I bought one e-bike from a company that said it was 95% assembled. I ended up having to pay a local bike mechanic $400 to fix what was wrong and assemble the rest.

Most online e-bikes will arrive at least partially assembled in a large box. You (or someone you hire) will need to attach the handlebars, front wheel, pedals, and often adjust brakes and gears. If not done correctly, this can be unsafe. For e-bikes, it also involves connecting electrical components, which adds another layer of complexity.

While a few online retailers offer "white glove" delivery or partner with local mechanics, this adds cost and complexity. In my research, it often leaves customers feeling like they paid more than they needed to for service that was sub-par.

The biggest con here is no test ride. This is a significant drawback. You won't know how the bike truly feels, fits, or handles until it arrives, assembled, at your door. There is one way to reduce the potential negative impact. Try to find a similar bike from the same manufacturer that you CAN test drive. At least you'll have some idea of what you are getting into. I did this with my Velotric Nomad II. I found a guy who lived nearby who had the Nomad, and that was more than good enough for me to know the bike would work for me.

One other con of online sales is lack of support in general. If you have a problem, you'll be dealing with customer service via phone or email, which can be less convenient than a face-to-face chat. That customer service team may be in a foreign country. It will be hard to hold the company accountable in these situations. Getting repairs or warranty work done can involve shipping parts (or even the whole bike) back, which can be a hassle.

If you choose to buy online

Look for detailed reviews from multiple sources, paying attention to comments on bike quality, assembly difficulty, and customer service experiences. Don't spend much time reading the reviews on the retailer's site. Instead, use third-party sources. Also, go to e-bike forums on social media and post questions about the company. Ask other riders what their experiences were. Take your time here. This is your opportunity to stop trouble before it starts.

Also understand the return policy before you buy. What are the costs? What is the timeframe? Is it easy to return a large item like an e-bike? Remember you will be expected to pack the bike in the original box and packing materials. You will have to figure out how to get this big, heavy box to the shipper. In almost all cases, you will be asked to pay a restocking fee which can vary between 10-35%.

Unless you know how to wrench your own bike, you will also need to budget for assembly. Budget both the money and the time it will take. Assess your own skillset. If you do have the skills and tools to do it, you might have no problem with assembly. Otherwise, you will need to hire a local mechanic, and will they work on a brand they don't sell?

Now is a good time to check and double check how the company handles warranty claims and technical support. Do they have service partners in your area? Will they ship you any parts you need free of charge, or will you have to pay shipping? Once again assess your mechanical skills and decide if you can make the repair on your own.

I don't want to make it sound like you cannot get a nice e-bike online or that you cannot get a good deal. I do want to make sure you are aware of the pitfalls.

My own experience leaves me scoring 50/50. I have purchased two e-bikes online. One simply didn't fit me, and I sold it at a big loss. The second was perfect and is my most beloved bike. Your mileage may literally vary.

Buying at big box stores

(Cautionary advice) You might see e-bikes for sale at large department stores or sporting goods chains. While the prices can seem attractive, I generally advise extreme caution when considering these options. I don't personally know of anyone who has been happy with their experience buying at a big box store.

Why? There are many compromises involved that you might not know exist until it's too late. To reach very low-price points, these e-bikes often use lower-grade components (brakes, gears, motors, batteries). This can lead to a less enjoyable riding experience, lower reliability, and potential safety issues. Sometimes, the big box stores offer older models. You may not be getting the bike you are seeing advertised everywhere else but instead, an older version of it.

Also note that bikes at big box stores are often assembled by general staff who may lack specialized bicycle or e-bike training. Improper assembly is a significant safety risk. I've heard many stories of bikes with loose handlebars, incorrectly installed brakes, or poorly tuned gears coming from these stores.

You will also find out that there is a complete lack of specialized support at these stores. Big box stores offer many products. They typically lack the expertise to offer meaningful advice, proper fitting, or after-sales service and repairs for e-bikes, which may be on the aisle between televisions and refrigerators. If something goes wrong, you'll likely be directed to a manufacturer's helpline rather than receiving local, hands-on assistance. While a big box store might seem convenient, the potential compromises in quality, safety, and support make them a risky choice for a significant purchase like an e-bike, especially when comfort, reliability, and peace of mind are paramount.

Choosing where to buy your e-bike is a key step. While online and big box stores have their place, the personalized service, expert assembly, crucial test rides, and ongoing support offered by a local bike shop make it, in my view, the clear winner and the highly recommended choice for senior riders venturing into the exciting world of electric cycling. My second choice would be a highly researched online purchase.

BONUS SECTION If you must buy online...

Navigating the online e-bike market can be exciting yet overwhelming, offering a vast selection but often requiring more research and some self-assembly. Many companies now blend online sales with physical showrooms or dealer networks. Here are some of the top and most noteworthy online e-bike retailers in the United States.

NOTE - I have purchased e-bikes from Velotric, and Lectric Bike Company online. I have purchased e-Bikes from Pedego at three different Pedego dealerships. I have also talked with close friends and relatives who purchased their e-bikes online and researched e-bikes in popular forums to compile this information. It is my best advice, but as always, your experience may vary.

Rad Power Bikes (https://www.radpowerbikes.com/)

As one of the pioneers and largest direct-to-consumer e-bike brands, Rad Power Bikes offers a comprehensive range of models for nearly every purpose, from rugged fat-tire adventures and utility-focused cargo bikes to approachable city commuters and convenient folding options.

Strengths. Extensive selection covering many niches, a large ecosystem of first-party accessories, strong brand recognition, competitive pricing, and a growing number of Rad Mobile Service vans and retail/service locations offering test rides and support in key areas.

Weaknesses. Due to their volume, customer service can sometimes experience delays. Reliance on some proprietary parts can occasionally complicate repairs at independent bike shops. Like most online brands, home assembly is standard unless a service option is chosen.

Lectric eBikes. (https://lectricebikes.com/)

Lectric has made a massive impact on the market with its focus on affordability, particularly with its flagship XP series of folding fat-tire e-bikes. They aim to make E-biking accessible through aggressive pricing and popular, practical designs.

Strengths. Industry-leading low prices, immense popularity (especially in the folding category), quick shipping, and an expanding lineup that now includes cargo, commuter, and trike models. They offer significant value for budget-conscious buyers.

Weaknesses. To achieve low costs, components are often basic, which may impact long-term durability or ride refinement for some users. Customer service and quality control can sometimes struggle to keep pace with rapid growth. Bikes can be heavy, and assembly/tuning are crucial. While their bikes tend to get good reviews, some reviewers question durability and quality.

SPECIAL NOTE: I purchased a bike online from Lectric eBikes. It was their trike. It was advertised as 95% assembled and ready to go but when it arrived it needed a lot of work. I also had to replace one wheel and fender because they were damaged in shipping. The company did send me replacement parts, but this took a couple of weeks. I ended up having to spend several hundred dollars to hire a local bike mechanic to get the bike in running order. It also didn't fit me very well. One of the hazards of buying online is that you cannot know for sure if the bike suits you until it arrives and then it's too late. Lectric sells a lot of bikes but for me, it wasn't a good experience. This was 18 months ago, and things could have changed since then. Just an FYI.

Aventon Bikes. (https://www.aventon.com/)

Aventon strikes a balance between value, style, and performance, often incorporating features like integrated batteries, torque sensors for a smoother ride, and app connectivity. They have also heavily invested in a dealer network alongside their online presence.

Strengths. Sleek, modern designs and good build quality for the price. The availability through numerous local bike shops is a major advantage, allowing customers to test ride, get professional assembly, and access local service – a significant benefit even when considering an online purchase.

Weaknesses. Prices are generally higher than budget leaders like Lectric. While the dealer network is a strength, it means online buyers might pay a bit more for that infrastructure. Some models are known for being heavy. My two friends who own Aventon bikes love them and believe that the slightly higher price compared to some of the bargain brands was a good investment.

Ride1Up (https://ride1up.com/)

Known for providing excellent "bang for your buck," Ride1Up often includes higher-quality components (like hydraulic brakes or advanced sensors) than expected at their price points. They cater to a variety of riders with commuter, gravel, cruiser, and moped-style options.

Strengths. Great value proposition, often featuring upgraded components. They have a strong reputation for U.S.-based customer support and offer a diverse range of styles, appealing to both performance-seekers and commuters.

Weaknesses. Primarily an online-only experience, limiting test rides and local support (unless you pay a local shop). Assembly is required, and as with any online purchase, there's a risk of shipping damage or minor out-of-the-box adjustments being needed.

Velotric. (https://www.velotricbike.com/)

Velotric has quickly gained attention by focusing on reliable, stylish, and user-friendly e-bikes, often emphasizing safety certifications like UL (Underwriters Laboratories) for their battery and electrical systems. They aim to provide a quality experience at a competitive mid-range price.

Strengths. Strong focus on safety (UL-certified), clean designs with integrated batteries, good balance of quality components and price, and generally positive reviews regarding ride comfort and customer support. They also have a growing network of local test-ride and service partners.

Weaknesses. As a relatively newer company, their long-term track record is still being established. While they have test-ride partners, their physical presence isn't as vast as Pedego or Aventon. Assembly is typically required for direct online orders.

SPECIAL NOTE. I purchased a bike online from Velotric called the Nomad II. I have to say it was a great experience. The bike came very well packed and is full of great features. I knew up front it was shipping at "85%" assembled. I arranged for my local bike mechanic (say hi to Joe again...) to assemble it and even though the company provides a quick-start guide, owner's manuals, and assembly videos that will walk you through the assembly, Joe said it was easy and didn't need to refer to the manufacturer's help guide. Since Joe is very experienced, this is something to keep in mind. Velotric bikes will require some assembly to ride but, in my opinion, the pain of assembly is well worth it. Velotric uses very high-quality components for the price point, and I simply love the Nomad II. It's the best e-bike I have ever ridden or tested. I will say that their warranty department stands behind the accessories they sell but may take a few days to respond whereas your local bike shop will be able to respond much sooner.

Pedego Electric Bikes. (https://pedegoelectricbikes.com/)

Pedego's primary strength and business model revolves around its extensive network of dedicated Pedego-branded local stores across the country. They focus on creating a fun, accessible e-biking experience with a wide variety of styles, often appealing to leisure riders and seniors.

Strengths. Unparalleled local dealer support, offering test rides, professional sales advice, assembly, and crucially, local servicing and warranty support. They foster a strong community feel and offer a wide range of comfortable, user-friendly designs. They offer bikes for all types of riders.

Weaknesses. Prices are generally noticeably higher than direct-to-consumer brands, reflecting the cost of their brick-and-mortar network. While you can browse and potentially initiate purchases online, their model heavily encourages (and is best experienced through) their local dealers.

Regarding the Pedego dealer network

Pedego's dealer network has shrunk in many areas. I used to live in the Seattle area. When I bought my first Pedego they had two dealers in Seattle, one in Tacoma one in Sequim and one in Richland, WA. As of this writing, all the Pedego dealers in Washington have closed. They do have many dealerships, but they aren't as widespread as they once were and many of you will need to buy their products direct, online.

SPECIAL NOTE. I have owned four Pedego e-bikes. In my opinion, they are generally good quality bikes, built to last. The four bikes I have owned were all expensive compared to the competition. Pedego bikes are typically a little heavy and offer a somewhat dated style. There's nothing flashy about most of their models. They are however a solid, meat and potatoes brand that you can usually count on. They have recently reduced prices to become more competitive and if you like their selection, I can tell you that you'll most likely be satisfied. You should know that several of their models have faced recalls and some lawsuits. I have never had any issues with any of my Pedego bikes. I have really enjoyed all four e-bikes I purchased from Pedego and I still ride my Pedego Fat-Tire Trike.

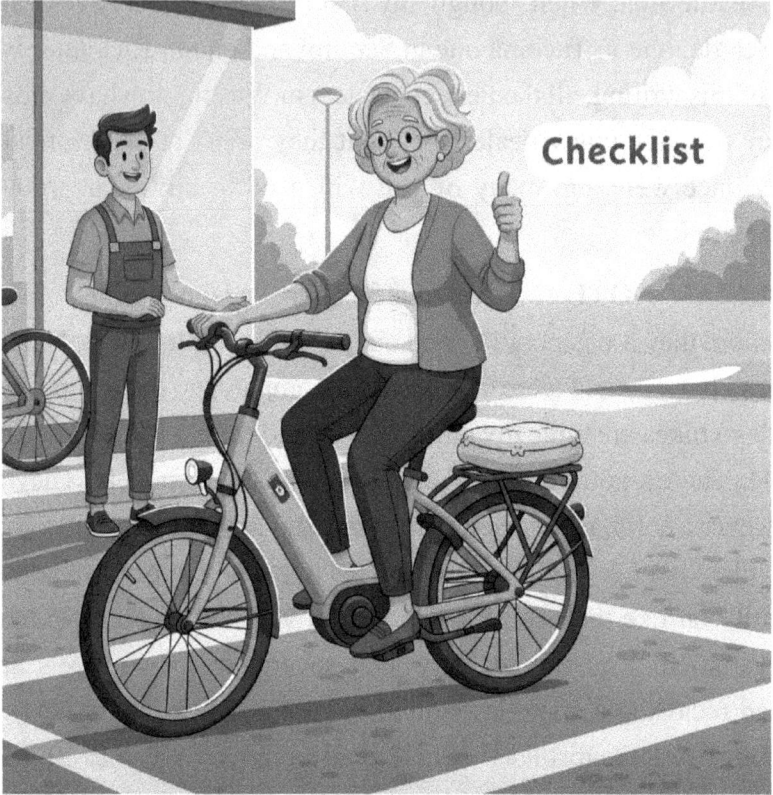

CHAPTER 7:
TEST RIDING LIKE A PRO

I've discussed test rides in previous chapters and now I want to devote an entire section of the book to test rides. I believe test rides are the most exciting and important step in your e-bike journey. Think of it like trying on a new pair of walking shoes; you wouldn't buy them without making sure they fit perfectly and feel comfortable, would you? An e-bike is an investment in your freedom, health, and enjoyment, so finding the one that feels like it was made just for you is paramount, especially for seniors. This chapter will offer an in-depth guide on how to make the most of your test rides, ensuring you choose an e-bike that you'll love and feel confident riding for years to come.

7.1. Why test riding is important

- Feeling the weight, balance and effects of the motor assist trumps reading reviews and looking at pictures. Nothing can replace the actual experience of riding an e-bike. This is your chance to truly feel the bike. Here's why a thorough test ride should be a priority.
- Can you comfortably manage the bike when you're not riding it? Try walking it a short distance.
- Does it feel manageable if you need to lift the front wheel slightly, perhaps to navigate a small curb (even if you plan to avoid them?)
- A bike that feels too cumbersome can be off-putting and even a safety concern.
- Is it easy to balance?

- How stable does the e-bike feel when you first get on?
- Pay attention to how it handles at very low speeds, such as when starting from a stop or making a tight turn in a shop's parking lot. A bike that feels wobbly or top-heavy might not be the right fit.
- Try the motor assist. This is where the magic of an e-bike comes in, but not all motor systems feel the same.
- How does the assistance engage when you start pedaling? Is it a smooth, gentle nudge, or does it feel more like a sudden surge? Most people prefer a smooth, intuitive assist.
- Try out the different levels of assistance. Can you easily switch between them? Does each level provide a noticeable and useful difference in power?
- Listen to the motor. Most are very quiet, but it's something to note.

A test ride allows you to answer these crucial questions based on your personal experience, not just what a brochure tells you.

7.2. What to pay attention to: Your test ride checklist

When you're out on your test ride, it's easy to get caught up in the fun and forget to check specific things. I've created a special checklist for you to help you stay on task.

Mounting and dismounting ease —This is a big one!

Can you get on and off the bike easily and safely? Consider a step-through frame (also called a low-step or easy-entry frame). These are incredibly popular with seniors as they don't require you to lift your leg high over the frame.

Check the stand over height. When you're standing still with the bike between your legs, is there enough clearance? You should be able to stand comfortably flat-footed over the bike, or very close to it.

Balance and stability at low speeds

As mentioned before, ride slowly. Try to maintain a straight line. Does it feel stable and controllable?

Practice starting and stopping a few times.

Good brakes are non-negotiable for safety.

Are the brake levers easy for your hands to reach and squeeze?

How do the brakes respond? They should feel powerful and bring you to a smooth, controlled stop without being overly sudden or "grabby."

Most quality e-bikes come with hydraulic disc brakes, which offer excellent stopping power in all weather conditions.

Motor engagement and smoothness of assist

Pedal and see how quickly and smoothly the motor kicks in. Does it feel natural?

When you stop pedaling, does the motor disengage promptly?

If there's a throttle (some e-bikes have them, allowing for motor power without pedaling), try it out to see how it responds.

Comfort of seat and handlebars

Comfort is king for enjoyable rides! Is the seat (sometimes called a saddle) comfortable, even for a short test ride? While saddles can often be swapped out, a good starting point is a plus. Look for wider, cushioned saddles if that's your preference.

Are the handlebars at a comfortable height and distance for you? Many seniors prefer a more upright riding posture, which is easier on the back and neck. Your arms should have a slight bend at the elbows.

Do the handlebar grips feel comfortable in your hands? Are they loose? Do they spin in place? Locking grips are best and don't move or spin.

Try shifting gears (you probably have to be riding the bike and using the pedals to do this). Even with motor assist, gears are important for tackling different terrains and maintaining a comfortable pedaling cadence.

How easy is it to shift gears? Are the shifters intuitive (e.g., thumb shifters, twist grips?) Do the gears change smoothly and quickly? Try shifting both up and down through the gears.

Don't be shy about asking to test ride a few different models if the first one doesn't feel quite right. The shop staff should be happy to help you find your perfect match. Also, don't necessarily trust your first impressions. Don't be in a rush. Try one bike, switch to another and then go back to the first bike. This gives you a better, more complete perspective.

7.3. Asking the right questions

Your test ride isn't just about how the bike feels. It's also your prime opportunity to ask the bike shop staff important questions. I've compiled a list of some of things you should ask.

Battery

Range. "What is the realistic range I can expect from this battery with my type of riding?" (Mention if you live in a hilly area or plan on using higher assist levels often).

Charging. "How long does the battery take to fully charge?" and "Is the battery easily removable for charging indoors?"

Lifespan & Replacement. "What is the expected lifespan of the battery, and roughly how much does a replacement cost?"

Warranty

"What does the warranty cover specifically – the frame, motor, battery, and other components?"

"How long is the warranty period for each of these key parts?" (Batteries and motors often have different warranty lengths than the frame).

"What is the process if I need to make a warranty claim?"

Service and Support

"Where can this e-bike be serviced?" and "Do you service the e-bikes you sell here at this shop?"

"How readily available are spare parts if needed down the line?" (This is especially important for proprietary motor or battery systems).

Accessories

"What accessories are included (e.g., lights, kickstand, bell)?"

"What useful accessories can be easily added?" (Think about racks for carrying groceries, fenders for wet weather, mirrors for visibility, or a more comfortable saddle if the stock one isn't perfect).

"How might adding these accessories affect the bike's weight or balance?"

Take notes if you need to. The more information you have, the more confident you'll be in your final decision.

A thorough test ride, armed with this knowledge, will empower you to choose an e-bike that not only meets your needs but also brings you immense joy and confidence on every ride. Don't rush the process, listen to your body, and ask plenty of questions. If something doesn't feel right – stop, inquire, check and if need be, start over. You get to decide when the time is right.

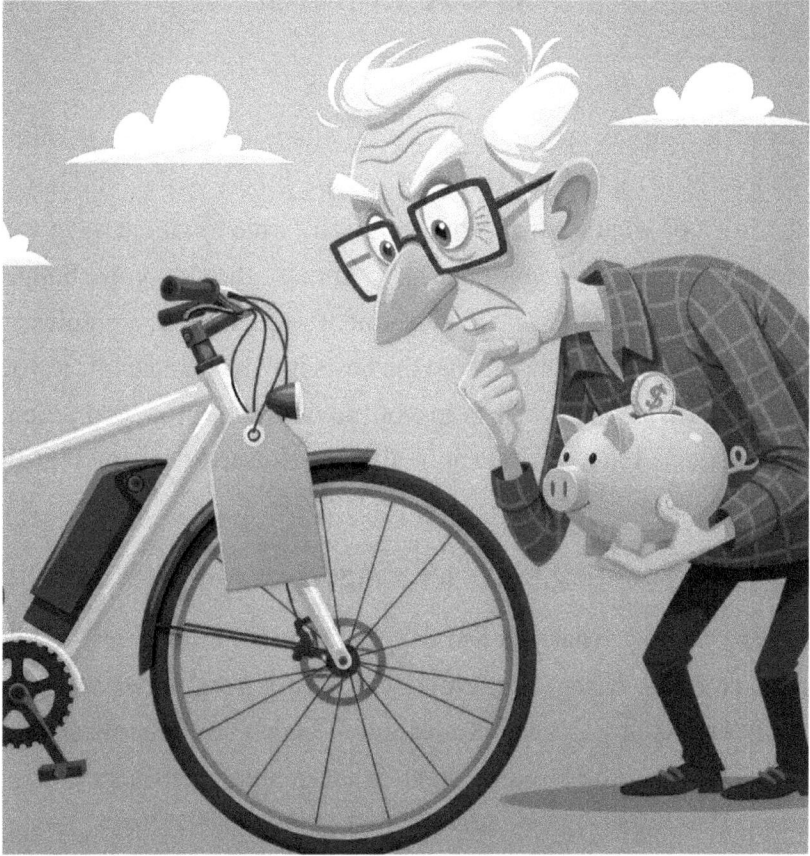

CHAPTER 8:
BUDGETING AND FINANCING
YOUR E-BIKE

Now that you've had the chance to either research your online purchase or complete a test ride of some e-bikes, you should have a better idea of what seems right for you. It's time to talk about a very practical decision—deciding how much should you budget. Purchasing an e-bike is an investment, and like any significant purchase, it's wise to understand the costs involved and explore your options. This chapter will help you navigate the financial side of buying your e-bike, so you can make an informed decision that fits your circumstances.

8.1. Understanding the price range

It's best to know what you can expect at certain price points. e-bike prices can vary quite a bit, typically ranging from under $1,000 to well over $5,000, and sometimes much higher for very specialized models. It's helpful to understand what generally influences these price differences:

Entry-level (roughly $800 - $1,500)

These bikes can be a good starting point. They usually feature basic hub motors (the motor is in the wheel hub) and simpler battery systems. Components like brakes and gears will be functional but may not be the most durable or refined.

Considerations. While more affordable, pay close attention to battery quality, (Is it UL listed? If not, I'd keep looking) motor reliability, and warranty terms. They might be heavier and have a shorter range. Good for casual, flatter rides.

Mid-range (roughly $1,500 - $3,000)

This is often the sweet spot for many seniors. All but two of the e-bikes I purchased fall into this price range. Here you'll find bikes with more reliable and smoother motor systems (including some mid-drive motors, which are located near the pedals and often provide a more natural feel). Batteries will generally be UL listed and have a longer range and lifespan. Components like brakes (often hydraulic disc brakes), gears, and suspension will be better quality, offering improved performance and durability. Frames might be lighter and offer better designs, including more refined step-through options.

Considerations. These bikes typically offer a great balance of quality, features, and price. They are well-suited for regular use, varied terrain, and longer rides.

Premium (Roughly $3,000 - $5,000+)

At this level, you're looking at top-tier components, advanced motor and battery technology (often lighter, more powerful, and with greater range), sophisticated suspension systems, and lighter, stronger frame materials. Features might include integrated lighting, advanced displays, and premium comfort elements.

Considerations. These are excellent bikes for avid riders, those tackling very challenging terrain, or anyone who wants the best performance and features. The investment is higher, but so is the quality and often the longevity.

Key factors influencing price

Motor type. Mid-drive motors (located at the crank set) are generally more expensive but offer better balance and a more intuitive riding feel than hub motors (located in the front or rear wheel hub).

Battery capacity and quality. Larger capacity (measured in Watt-hours or Wh) means longer range. Higher quality cells (from brands like Samsung, LG, Panasonic) usually mean longer lifespan and better performance. Batteries that are UL listed will add more cost.

Component quality. Brakes, gears (derailleurs), suspension, tires, and even saddles and grips contribute to the price. Better components mean smoother operation, greater durability, and enhanced safety.

Frame material and design. Lightweight aluminum alloys are common. Carbon fiber frames are lighter and stronger but significantly more expensive. The complexity of the frame design (e.g., sophisticated step-throughs) also plays a role.

Brand reputation and warranty. Established brands often invest more in research, development, and customer support, which can be reflected in the price. A good warranty provides peace of mind.

Think about your needs and how often you plan to ride. It's not always necessary to buy the most expensive option, but investing in a quality e-bike that meets your specific requirements will likely lead to a more enjoyable and lasting experience.

8.2. Additional costs: accessories, maintenance, and insurance

When budgeting for your e-bike, it's important to look beyond the initial purchase price. There are a few other potential costs to consider:

Start with the essential accessories

Helmet. Non-negotiable for safety. Budget $40 - $100+ for a good quality, comfortable helmet.

Buy a lock. A sturdy U-lock or heavy-duty chain lock is crucial to protect your investment. Expect to spend $50 - $150+.

If your bike doesn't come with integrated lights, you'll need to buy at least one front light. If you want brighter lights for better visibility, budget for front and rear lights ($30 - $100+.)

You'll need a bell or a horn. In some jurisdictions it's a legal requirement. Even if it's not legally required, it just makes sense to get one. These are essential for alerting pedestrians and other cyclists. They also help foster good biking manners and don't cost very much. Available under $15.

You will need to get either an air compressor or a floor pump for home and a small portable pump for on-the-go adjustments. Budget $20-$120.

Comfort and convenience accessories (optional but often desired)

Fenders/mudguards. Keep you cleaner in wet conditions.

Rack and panniers/basket. For carrying groceries, a bag, or other items.

Mirror. Improves awareness of traffic behind you. (Required in some jurisdictions.)

More comfortable saddle or grips. If the stock ones aren't to your liking.

Water bottle cage. To stay hydrated.

You will also need to budget for regular maintenance. Like any bicycle, an e-bike requires regular maintenance to keep it running smoothly and safely.

Tune-ups. Plan for a professional tune-up annually or every 1,000-1,500 miles. This might cost $75 - $250, depending on where you live and the complexity of your bike.

Brake pads. Will wear out and need replacing.

Tires. May need replacing due to wear or punctures (though good quality tires and liners like Tannus Armour, as discussed elsewhere in this book, can minimize this). Unless you ride often, you probably won't have to replace a tire unless you suffer tire damage from a crash or a blow-out.

Chain and cassette. These drivetrain components wear over time and will eventually need replacement. However, it's unlikely you will have to deal with this for several years.

Battery care. While also not a frequent cost, batteries have a finite lifespan (typically 3-5 years or a certain number of charge cycles). A replacement battery can cost several hundred to over $1,000, so it's good to be aware of this long-term expense. If you do replace your battery, make sure it is with a manufacturer's approved battery and look for one that is UL listed.

Another expense you may incur relates to insurance. Not all e-bike owners want or need insurance, but if you decide you couldn't afford to replace your e-bike if stolen, consider insurance a priority.

Homeowners/renters insurance. Check if your current policy covers e-bikes, especially for theft. There might be limits on value.

Specialized e-bike insurance. Several companies offer specific e-bike insurance that can cover theft, damage, and even liability. This might be worth considering, especially for more expensive e-bikes.

Factoring these additional costs into your budget from the outset will help you avoid surprises down the road.

8.3. Financing

If paying the full price of an e-bike upfront isn't feasible or desirable, there are often financing options available. If you buy your e-bike at a local bike shop, the shop may partner with financing companies (like Klarna, Affirm, or Synchrony Financial) to offer payment plans.

You apply for credit through the store, and if approved, you can pay for the e-bike in monthly instalments over a set period (e.g., 6, 12, or 24 months).

These plans are convenient, often with promotional offers like 0% interest for a limited time if paid within that period. It's extremely important that you pay strict attention to the terms of these loans—especially if they're zero-interest loans that must be paid by a certain date. If you pay off 99% of the e-bike on time but miss the last payment, then you get a bill for high Interest rates that accrues from day one of the loan.

If you don't qualify for promotional rates, you should probably try your bank or apply for a new credit card that has low interest for a fixed time. Whatever plan you choose, be sure to read all the terms and conditions carefully.

As for the bank option, you could obtain a personal loan from your bank or a credit union. If you meet their income and credit score requirements, you borrow a lump sum and repay it in fixed monthly instillments over an agreed term, with interest.

Depending on your local lender, these plans can sometimes offer lower interest rates than store financing, especially if you have a good credit history. The downside here is that this decision will require a separate application process with a financial institution. That will add time to the equation and means you won't get your bike right away.

I suggest using a credit card as a last-ditch option. Most credit cards have a high interest rate but as I said, if you can get a new card with an introductory 0% APR offer it may be a good idea. This is very simple if you do already have a low-interest card but if not, it will be extra legwork to find a good deal and be aware...card interest rates can be very high if you carry a balance beyond any promotional period.

Important considerations for financing—Summary

- **Interest rates.** Understand the Annual Percentage Rate (APR) you'll be paying.
- **Loan term.** A longer term means lower monthly payments but more interest paid overall.
- **Fees.** Are there any origination fees or other charges?
- **Your budget.** Ensure the monthly payments fit comfortably within your budget.
- **Fine print.** Read everything before you sign. Be deliberate and do your research. If you commit to a long-term contract that you can't afford or that offers you less than fair terms, you won't enjoy your e-bike.

It's wise to only finance an amount you are confident you can repay without financial strain.

8.4. Government incentives/rebates

Federal e-bike incentives

As of mid-2025, there is no active federal tax credit or rebate program for e-bike purchases in the United States. The "Electric Bicycle Incentive Kickstart for the Environment (E-BIKE) Act" has been proposed in Congress. If it were to pass, it would offer a tax credit of 30% of the purchase price of a new e-bike, with a maximum credit of $1,500. However, it is crucial to understand that this is currently just a proposal and not law. You should monitor official government and news sources for any updates on this potential federal incentive.

In the current political climate at the time I wrote this book, it's highly unlikely the federal government will participate in any sort of grant or rebate programs for any type of electric vehicle, even if it's just a bicycle.

State-level e-bike rebate programs

Several states have implemented their own e-bike incentive programs. These vary significantly in terms of the rebate amount, eligibility criteria, and application process.

California: The California E-bike Incentive Project provides rebates to income-qualified residents. These can be up to $2,000. To qualify, residents generally need to have a household income at or below 300% of the federal poverty level. The program operates through specific application windows, which you'll need to monitor.

Colorado: Colorado offers a point-of-sale tax credit for all residents that provides an instant discount of $450 at participating retailers. There are no income restrictions for this base credit.

Connecticut: The Connecticut E-Bike Incentive Program offers rebates starting at $250. For low-income families, this amount can increase to $500.

Minnesota: Minnesota provides a rebate that covers 50-75% of the cost of an e-bike, up to a maximum of $1,500. The specific rebate amount is tiered based on the applicant's income.

Washington: The state of Washington offers an e-bike rebate program with a standard rebate of $300 for all residents. For those who meet low-income requirements, the rebate increases to $1,200.

Washington, D.C.: The District of Columbia has a voucher program that can provide up to $2,000 for the purchase of a cargo e-bike for low-income residents.

I live in Las Cruces, NM and our local utility offers up to $1,300 (half price) of an e-bike depending on income, and $900 to anyone who is in their service area, has an account, and buys a qualifying e-bike. I wasn't counting on that money but was happy to get it.

Other states with various e-bike incentive programs include Arizona, Florida (sales tax exemption), and Texas. It is always best to check your state's official government website for the most current information on available programs.

How to find and apply for e-bike rebates

To find and apply for these rebates, you should start by visiting the official websites of your state's department of transportation or energy office. You can also search online for "[Your State] e-bike rebate" or "[Your City] e-bike incentive." For local programs, check the website of your electricity provider.

When you find a program, be sure to carefully read the eligibility requirements, which often include residency, income level, and the type of e-bike that qualifies. Many programs require you to purchase your e-bike from a participating local retailer. You will typically need to provide proof of residency, and for income-qualified programs, proof of income. Some rebates are applied at the point of sale, while others require you to apply with your receipt after the purchase. Due to high demand, funding for these programs can be limited, so it is often advantageous to apply as soon as a program opens.

While not guaranteed, finding an applicable rebate or incentive could significantly reduce the overall cost of your new e-bike.

By carefully considering the price points, potential additional costs, and available financing or incentive programs, you can create a realistic budget for your e-bike purchase. This thoughtful approach will help ensure that your new e-bike brings you joy and freedom without causing financial stress.

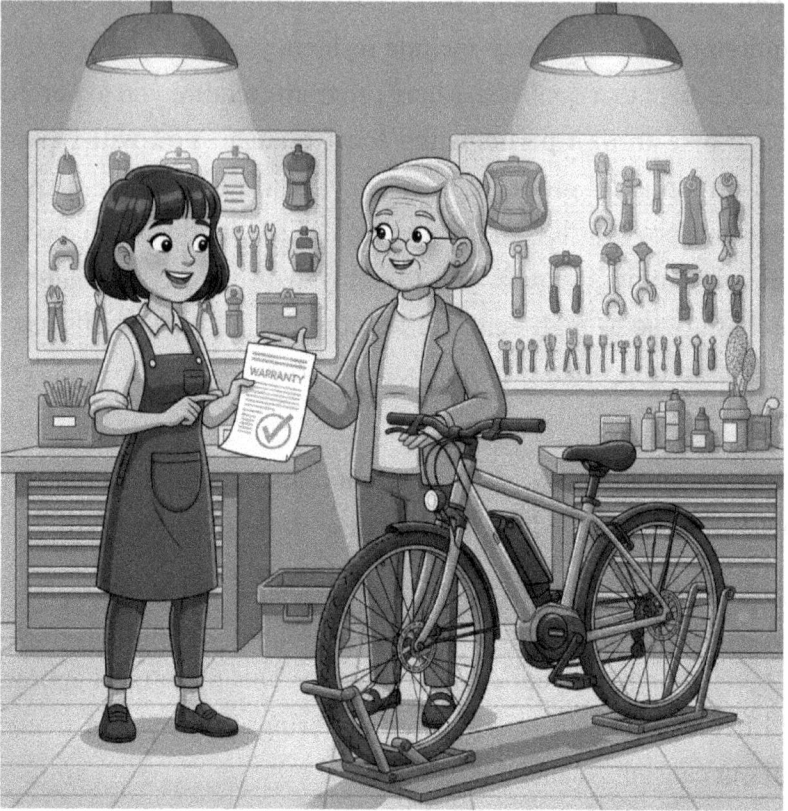

CHAPTER 9:
WARRANTIES, RETURNS, AND AFTER-SALE SUPPORT

Congratulations! Choosing and purchasing an e-bike is a major step. But your journey with the seller doesn't end when you hand over your payment. Understanding what happens after the sale is crucial for long-term satisfaction and peace of mind. A good warranty, a fair return policy, and accessible support can make all the difference, ensuring your investment is protected and you have help when you need it. Let's look at these important post-purchase considerations.

9.1. Understanding your warranty

Think of a warranty as the manufacturer's promise about the quality of their product and their commitment to fix certain issues within a specific timeframe. E-bike warranties usually cover different parts for different lengths of time, so it's essential to read the details carefully before you buy.

Here's a typical breakdown:

- **Frame.** The frame is the backbone of your e-bike, and manufacturers often show confidence here with longer warranty periods. It's common to see warranties ranging from five years to a lifetime for the frame, usually covering manufacturing defects rather than damage from accidents or misuse.
- **Motor.** The electric motor is a key component. Warranties for the motor (and often the associated electronic controller)

typically range from one to three years. These usually cover internal failures or malfunctions, not issues caused by water damage (unless specifically rated for it) or tampering.

- **Battery.** The battery is one of the most expensive parts of an e-bike. Most manufacturers offer a one to two-year warranty on the battery. This generally covers manufacturing defects and often guarantees a certain percentage of its original capacity after a set number of charge cycles or years. Battery warranties rarely cover degradation due to improper charging, storage, or physical damage.

- **Other components.** Parts like brakes, gears, handlebars, seats, and tires (often called "wear-and-tear" items) usually have a shorter warranty, often one year or sometimes only covering initial defects found within the first few rides. Some high-end components might carry their own manufacturer's warranty.

And here are key things to look for

Understand what is covered and, just as importantly, what isn't. Warranties usually exclude normal wear and tear, damage from accidents, improper assembly (a big reason I recommend local bike shops), or unauthorized modifications.

Do you need to register your e-bike online to activate the warranty? Depending on the state you live in, you just very well might need to do that. Make sure you do this promptly if required. Also see if the warranty can be transferred if you decide to sell the bike later. Most are non-transferable but I have purchased a few e-bikes where the warranty could transfer once.

Learn how you can make a claim. You may need to go through the shop where you bought the bike or deal directly with the manufacturer. Always read the fine print!

9.2. Return policies

Sometimes, despite all your research and even a test ride, you might find that the e-bike you bought just isn't the right fit. This is where the return policy comes in.

Policies vary, but many local bike shops offer a limited window (perhaps 7-14 days), where you might be able to exchange the bike or return it, often for store credit. Expect that if you've ridden it significantly, a full refund might not be possible, or a "re-stocking fee" might apply. The advantage here is that you can discuss the issue face-to-face.

If you bought the bike from an online retailer the process can be trickier. Most reputable online sellers have a return window (often 14-30 days), but you must read their policy carefully. The bike usually needs to be in "like new" condition. There are almost always re-stocking fees. Many online retailers charge a significant fee (sometimes 10-25% or more) for returns. You will almost certainly have to pay for the return shipping, which for a large, heavy box containing an e-bike can be very expensive (hundreds of dollars).

You will also be responsible for packaging. You'll need to repackage the bike securely in its original box, which can be challenging. I always encourage people to use a camera to make still photos or even videos of the unboxing process. This way, if you need to repack the bike, you have a reference to how each portion of the bike was prepared for a box.

The takeaway here is simple. Returning an e-bike, especially one bought online, can be costly and inconvenient. This underscores the importance of choosing carefully and, if possible, test-riding before you buy. I have always had a test ride of either the exact bike I want to buy or one that is similar. This greatly reduces the chance of a return.

9.3. Service and maintenance plans

Like a car, your e-bike needs regular check-ups and maintenance to run smoothly and safely. This is another area where your local bike shop truly shines.

Most bike shops include a free first tune-up (often after 30-90 days or a certain number of miles). This is important because new bikes often "settle in," and cables can stretch, requiring adjustments to brakes and gears. After the initial tune-up and check, you'll still need to consider ongoing maintenance. Your local bike shop can perform routine maintenance like brake adjustments, gear tuning, chain cleaning and lubrication, tire checks, and software updates for the e-bike system.

Some shops offer pre-paid service plans or packages, which can be a cost-effective way to cover your maintenance needs for a year or more. Ask if these are available and what they cover. Carefully check online reviews to see if the shop does a good job honoring the service plan.

When things go wrong, especially with the electrical components, having a trusted, trained mechanic nearby is invaluable. They have the diagnostic tools, spare parts (or access to them), and expertise to handle e-bike-specific issues. Even if you buy online, it's worth building a relationship with a local shop that is willing to work on your brand of e-bike (be aware that some shops may only service brands they sell). Regular, professional service is key to enjoying your e-bike safely for many years.

I am very lucky to have found the best bike mechanic in my small town. He takes total care of my two e-bikes and without him, I wouldn't have near as much peace of mind regarding the condition of my bikes. He's worth every penny I pay him.

Some of you may have sufficient mechanical skill to do your own repair. If so, I envy you. But based on my research, especially when it comes to the more complex e-bike, it still might be best to turn to a professional.

Understanding these post-purchase supports provides confidence in your investment. But the most important part of owning an es-bike is enjoying it safely. In my final part of the book, I turn my attention to the crucial topic of staying safe while you ride.

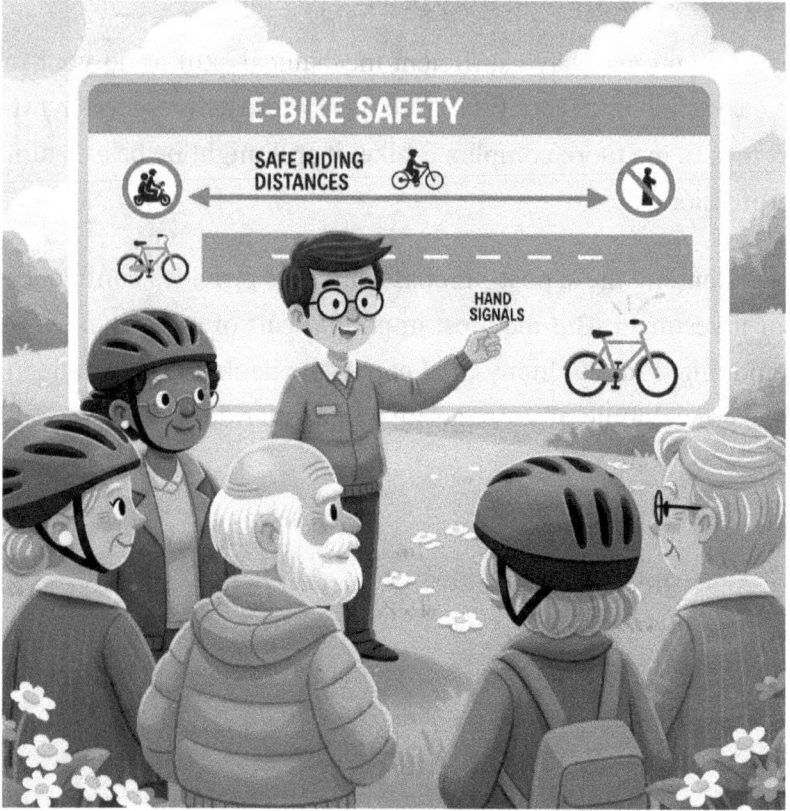

CHAPTER 10:
ESSENTIAL SAFETY GEAR FOR E-BIKE RIDERS

Just as you wouldn't drive a car without a seatbelt, certain gear is fundamental to safe cycling. Think of these items not as optional extras, but as part of your standard riding attire. They protect you, make you more visible to others, and enhance your comfort on every ride.

NOTE: In the appendices, I have a section devoted to my personal list of favorite accessories. The items on that list are items I use myself and that I bought and paid for with my own money, so you can know my recommendation of these items is sincere. In addition to that list, I have some basic items to consider.

10.1. Helmets

There's a good reason that I've mentioned bicycle helmets several times in this book. Wearing a helmet every time you ride should be standard operating procedure. Your brain is your most precious asset, and a fall can happen to anyone, anytime, regardless of experience or speed. E-bikes often travel at higher average speeds than traditional bikes, making head protection even more critical.

There are different types of helmets, and I believe there is a helmet for everyone. While any standard bicycle helmet is far better than none, consider looking at helmets specifically rated for e-bike use (often designated by the NTA 8776 standard). These are designed to provide protection at slightly higher impact speeds, common with e-bikes. Many helmets also offer features like Multi-directional

Impact Protection System (MIPS), designed to reduce rotational forces during a crash. Some even have built-in lights. Choose one with good ventilation for comfort.

Another crucial factor in selecting a helmet is finding one that fits. A helmet only works if it fits correctly. It should sit level on your head (not tilted back), covering your forehead. It should feel snug but not tight – you shouldn't be able to easily rock it back and forth or side to side. The "V" straps should meet just below your ears, and the chin strap should be snug enough that you can fit only one or two fingers between the strap and your chin. Try several models on in a shop to find one that feels right. If it doesn't fit properly or is uncomfortable, you won't wear it and that could be a very costly mistake.

Look for a helmet with professional certifications. Ensure your helmet meets safety standards. In the US, look for a CPSC (Consumer Product Safety Commission) sticker. In Canada, look for CSA, CPSC, Snell, or ASTM certifications.

Also, I'll mention MIPS again. A MIPS helmet will often provide the best protection for the money.

Here's something you might not know about helmets. They need to be replaced every three to five years. And if you drop your helmet on the concrete floor, or you have a crash, always replace your helmet. You need to replace it after any impact, even if it looks undamaged. The protective foam is designed to crush during one impact. It stops working once that happens.

10.2. Lights

Being seen is as important as seeing, especially on an e-bike. Lights are crucial, not just at night but during the day too. Many e-bikes come with integrated lights, but if your bike doesn't, or if you want extra visibility, invest in a good pair of lights.

You should have (at a minimum) a good front light which should be white. Most states require a light for night riding. And most states require that any light on the front of the bike should show white.

In addition to having this light to meet legal requirements, this front light helps you see the path ahead in low light and, crucially, makes you much more visible to oncoming traffic and pedestrians during the day.

On all my bikes, I am lucky that the manufacturer included a white front headlight. But I take it a step further. Near the front headlight, I mount a second USB-powered blinking, LED (white) light. A blinking light is much easier to see and can make a difference between being seen or not seen. These lights are available at places like Amazon for as little as $10.

You should also consider having a rear, red light. This is vital for ensuring traffic approaching from behind can see you clearly. Many rear lights have flashing modes.

As with the front light, both my e-bikes have red rear taillights and again, I add a rear LED flashing light. Be sure to check the laws in your area that govern bicycles and e-bikes because there may be certain requirements or restrictions that should guide your decisions here.

To sum up the lighting section, be sure to have both day and night visibility. Modern, bright LED lights are highly effective even in bright daylight. Using a flashing light during the day significantly increases your chances of being noticed by drivers.

For night riding, a steady front beam helps you see, while a flashing rear light demands attention. Look for lights with good side visibility too.

10.3. Reflective clothing and gear

While lights send out beams, reflective materials bounce light back towards its source, making you appear brightly illuminated when caught in headlights.

Brightly colored clothing (like neon yellow, green, or orange) is excellent for daytime visibility. For dawn, dusk, and nighttime riding, incorporate reflective elements. This could be a lightweight vest, ankle bands (which are very effective due to their motion), reflective stripes on jackets or pants, or even reflective tape applied to your helmet or bike frame. The more points of reflection you have, the more easily a driver can recognize you as a cyclist.

Personal note – I wear a construction-type vest and look like a member of the Village People when I ride – but people can see me. That's all that matters.

You can buy inexpensive reflective stickers at Amazon for about $5. Apply them to your bike, clothing, helmet, etc. If you ride at night. Also make sure any accessories you buy have reflective strips attached. Saddle bags, tank bags, etc. should always have reflective parts.

10.4. Gloves

Cycling gloves might seem minor, but they serve important purposes for senior riders including added comfort and protection.

Comfort: Padded cycling gloves help absorb vibrations from the handlebars, reducing pressure on your palms and wrists. This can prevent numbness and discomfort, especially on longer rides.

Protection: In the unfortunate event of a fall, our instinct is to put our hands out. Gloves provide a crucial layer of protection against scrapes and cuts, saving your palms from painful "road rash." They come in half-finger (good for warm weather and dexterity) and full-finger (more protection, better for cool weather) styles.

My advice is to not penny-pinch here. I consider my riding gloves to be the most important piece of safety gear after my helmet and reflective vest.

10.5. Eyewear

Protecting your eyes is essential for both comfort and clear vision while riding.

Cycling eyewear shields your eyes from wind (which can cause tearing and obscure vision), dust, grit kicked up by cars, and insects. This is especially important at e-bike speeds.

If you have sunglasses that may be good enough. There are special sunglasses designed for cycling that reduce glare and protect your eyes from harmful UV rays. Many offer interchangeable lenses, allowing you to swap between dark lenses for bright sun, amber or rose lenses for enhancing contrast in overcast conditions, and clear lenses for night riding or low light. Look for styles that offer good coverage and don't obstruct your peripheral vision.

In my case, my prescription sunglasses came with the same features as specialized riding glasses, so I didn't do anything special here.

What's important is to always have SOMETHING shielding your eyes. If you're going 20 MPH and an insect smacks you in the eye – you'll understand why glasses matter.

Investing in this essential gear is an investment in your safety and enjoyment. When you feel protected and visible, you can ride with greater confidence, allowing you to fully embrace the freedom your e-bike offers.

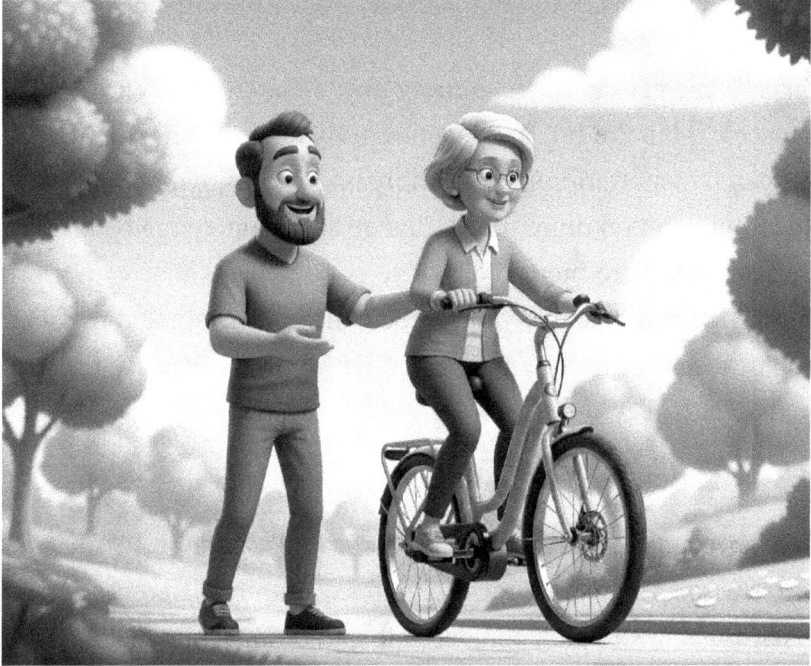

CHAPTER 11:
SAFE RIDING TIPS FOR 55+ E-BIKE RIDERS

This is a chapter dedicated entirely to your safety and confidence on your new e-bike! e-bikes are wonderfully empowering, but like any mode of transport, riding them safely is key to enjoyment. As we get older, our reaction times might change and maintaining balance can sometimes require more focus. The good news is that with a little knowledge and practice, you can become a very safe and proficient e-bike rider. This chapter is packed with tips specifically for riders aged 55 and over.

11.1. Starting and stopping safely

Getting used to the assist. The motor assist on an e-bike is what makes it so special, but it also requires a slightly different approach to starting and stopping compared to a traditional bicycle.

Before you start

When you're first getting used to your e-bike, or if you're in a crowded area, always start with the motor assist on the lowest setting (or even off). This prevents any unexpected surges of power.

Have at least one foot firmly on the ground before you start pedaling. I also strongly suggest you grab one of the hand brakes before and as you mount the bike. This stops the bike from rolling out from underneath you.

Always check your surroundings. Also look around for pedestrians, traffic, or obstacles before you set off.

Starting smoothly

Begin with a gentle push on the pedals. The motor will engage smoothly, especially on lower assist levels. Avoid stomping hard on the pedals right away. After you get to using the throttle (if your bike has a throttle) you may want to do what I do which is use the throttle on low power to take off and then begin to pedal. It makes for a more confident and smooth start.

Be ready for that little bit of extra "oomph" when the motor kicks in. It's a pleasant feeling once you're used to it! It can be described as a nudge. I only mention it here because it may catch you by surprise the first time you ride out. After that it won't even register.

Find a quiet, open space like an empty parking lot or a park path to practice starting and stopping until it feels second nature. Avoid crowds and traffic during this stage of your "training." Give yourself room and time to succeed. Remember, this is supposed to be fun!

Stopping safely

Before you apply the brakes, stop pedaling. This tells the motor to disengage. Remember if the bike doesn't have forward momentum you have to be able to put your feet down to balance it.

I'll cover braking in more detail shortly, but always aim for smooth, controlled stops. Apply the brakes smoothly and gently. Don't grab them.

As you come to a stop, prepare to put one foot down to maintain balance. Choose the side that feels most comfortable and stable for you. You may be starting to see why I so strongly recommend a step-through e-bike for senior riders. It's much easier to dismount as well as mount.

When you've stopped for more than a few seconds (e.g., at a traffic light), some riders like to turn the assist level to 'off' as an extra precaution against accidental engagement. There is no right or wrong way to do this. I personally leave PAS on but in the lowest setting in case I need throttle to launch. Try it both ways and pick the way that feels comfortable to you.

11.2. Managing Speed

Using pedal assist levels wisely

Your w-bike can likely go faster than you might be used to on a regular bicycle, especially with higher assist levels. Managing your speed is crucial for safety.

Familiarize yourself with what each pedal assist level does. Start at one and work your way up. Most e-bikes go from one to five.

Set your overall power levels to a gentler setting (e.g., Eco, 1-2): Provide gentle assistance, ideal for flat ground, conserving battery, or when you want more of a workout. This is best for starting out and in busy areas.

Medium levels (e.g., Tour, Normal, 3): Offer a good balance of assistance and battery life. Great for general riding and small hills.

High levels (e.g., Sport, Turbo, 4-5): Provide significant power for tackling steep hills or getting a quick boost. Use these judiciously as they drain the battery faster and can make the bike feel very quick.

Match speed to conditions

Slow down in busy areas. Always reduce your speed and assist level around pedestrians, other cyclists, or in areas with potential hazards.

Be very careful on downhill grades. E-bikes are heavier than traditional bikes, which means they can pick up speed quickly downhill. Use lower gears and rely on your brakes, not just the motor being off.

If you're riding on roads or paths with posted speed limits, adhere to them. They apply to you even as an e-biker.

While it's tempting to use the highest assist level all the time, it's often safer (and better for your fitness and battery range) to use the lowest assist level that allows you to pedal comfortably. Start low and work your way up to the higher PAS when and if you need it.

11.3. Braking techniques

Using both brakes

Your e-bike's brakes are powerful and knowing how to use them effectively is essential. Most e-bikes have two brake levers: one for the front brake and one for the rear.

For maximum stopping power and control, always aim to use both brakes simultaneously and evenly.

Using only the rear brake can cause a skid, and applying only the front brake too hard can, in extreme cases, cause the rear wheel to lift or even send you over the handlebars (though this is less common with the weight distribution of e-bikes).

Practice feathering both brakes gently to scrub off speed or come to a smooth stop.

Look ahead! Don't wait until the last second to brake. Anticipate your stops and slow down a little earlier than you would have on a traditional bicycle.

Scan the path or road for potential hazards, traffic lights, stop signs, or pedestrians who might step out.

Start braking earlier and more gently than you think you might need to, especially in wet or slippery conditions. This gives you more time to react if something unexpected happens.

Avoid grabbing a handful of brake lever suddenly. Instead, squeeze the levers gently, and progressively. The harder you squeeze, the more braking power you'll get.

When braking hard, especially downhill, shift your weight slightly backward on the saddle. This helps maintain traction and stability.

In your safe practice area, try a few harder (but still controlled) stops to get a feel for how your brakes respond in an urgent situation. Practice worse-case scenarios when the pressure is not on. That way, if you ever need to apply brakes in an emergency, you'll be more ready.

11.4. Riding in traffic and on trails

Rules of the road, trail etiquette

Whether you're on city streets or park trails, knowing the rules and expected behaviors keeps everyone safer and happier.

Be visible when you are riding in traffic, or on or near roads or streets. Wear bright clothing. Ensure your lights are on, especially in dim conditions or at night. Make sure you have reflectors on your bicycle in addition to lighting. They are inexpensive and readily available.

Obey all traffic signals, stop signs, and road markings, just as you would in a car. In most jurisdictions, you can be cited for violating traffic laws on a bicycle just like you can in a car. It's also polite, safe, and is common sense to follow the rules. Like it or not, every one of us is an ambassador for e-biking. Our conduct is judged by those who are around us.

Please ride predictably. Ride in a straight line and avoid sudden swerving. This is because you never know who's coming up behind you, and if you are unpredictable in your path, you could accidentally cause a collision.

Claim your lane when necessary

If a lane is too narrow for a car to pass you safely within the lane, it's often safer to "take the lane" by riding closer to the center of it. This discourages unsafe passes. However, be mindful of holding up traffic and pull over to let cars pass when it's safe to do so.

If there's a designated bike lane, use it. It will always be safer and makes your path more predictable for cars and others traveling on the same road.

When riding past parked cars, leave enough space to avoid a suddenly opened door.

Riding on multi-use trails/paths

Remember these paths are often shared with pedestrians, joggers, dog walkers, and other cyclists. Give way when it's appropriate and when you can safely do so.

Do watch your speed. Travel at a speed that is safe and courteous for all users. I tend to always slow down when passing a pedestrian because I do not want to alarm or startle them. It's easy enough to speed back up once you're down the trail.

Alert others before passing (see "Communication" below). Pass on the left and give plenty of room. I always tap my bell and say out loud "On your left" to make sure the person in front of me is aware of my presence and is not alarmed when I come up behind them.

Generally, keep to the right side of the path unless passing. This makes it easy for everyone to have room to roam.

Approach dogs slowly and be aware they might be on a leash or could move unexpectedly. If you see a dog that is NOT on a leash, my best advice is to turn around and go the other way. Dogs are known to chase bicycles based on a simple prey response they have inherited through their wolf DNA. There's no reason to tempt them.

Stay on marked trails to protect vegetation and wildlife. If you ride an e-bike and are seen trampling on nature, you can bet you will be reported and you will also denigrate the reputation of e-bikers.

11.5. Situational Awareness

Looking out for hazards, pedestrians, and other vehicles

Situational awareness simply means being constantly aware of what's happening around you. This is perhaps the most critical skill for safe riding.

Keep your head on a swivel. Don't just stare at the wheel in front of you. Keep your head up and scan your surroundings—ahead, to the sides, and even briefly behind you (or use a mirror).

Look for road hazards such as potholes, cracks, loose gravel, wet leaves, drain grates. Trash on the road can cause more problems than you might suspect.

Watch for pedestrians especially near crosswalks, bus stops, or in busy areas. Be aware they might be distracted (e.g., on their phones.) My approach is to always assume that the pedestrian doesn't see me, so it's my job to act accordingly.

Pay strict attention to cars, buses, motorcycles, and other cyclists. Try to anticipate their movements. Make eye contact with drivers when possible to ensure they've seen you. As I do with pedestrians, I always assume nearby vehicles do NOT see me and I ride defensively.

If you pay attention to anything I say in this chapter, make sure it's this. Be extra cautious at intersections. This is where most car-bicycle collisions occur. A common occurrence is for a car to roll through the stop sign, into the crosswalk, and then they stop, look for traffic and go. If you're in that crosswalk when all this happens, you have a problem. Also, in North America, when you are coming up to an intersection, check your left mirror to see what's coming up from behind you. That car may be turning right in front of you so be prepared.

Your ears can also provide important clues. Listen for approaching vehicles, shouts, or other sounds that might indicate a potential hazard. Avoid wearing headphones that block out ambient noise. I use Apple Airpods which allow me to hear the music AND the ambient noise around me.

Always expect the unexpected. Assume that others may not see you or might make mistakes.

11.6. Communication

Clear communication with other road and trail users is vital for preventing accidents and misunderstandings. Use hand signals to indicate your intentions. The same standard hand signals used while operating a motor vehicle or motorcycle can be used on a bike.

Left turn: Extend your left arm straight out to the side.

Right turn: Extend your right arm straight out to the side OR extend your left arm out and bend it upwards at a 90-degree angle at the elbow (the traditional signal).

Stopping and slowing: Extend your left arm out and bend it downwards at a 90-degree angle at the elbow, with your palm facing backward.

Signal well in advance of your next turn or stop.

NOTE: Some e-bikes come with electronic turn signals. Both of my e-bikes offer this feature. They also include brake lights like the ones you find on cars. I use these instead of hand signals.

Using your bell and/or voice

Give a friendly ring of your bell (or a polite "Excuse me!" or "Passing on your left!") well in advance when approaching pedestrians from behind on a shared path.

A bell or horn can also be useful for alerting other cyclists.

Don't overuse these tools aggressively. A polite warning is usually sufficient. Your goal should merely be to alert the other person to your presence.

11.7. Riding with others:

Keeping pace, group etiquette

Riding with friends or in a group can be a wonderful social experience. Here are a few tips for group riding. Always communicate. Before you set off, discuss the route, planned pace, and any planned stops.

Ride at a comfortable pace—for you and for the group. If you're a stronger rider, be prepared to slow down for others. If you're slower, don't feel pressured to keep up beyond your comfort level. The group should accommodate the pace of its steadiest rider. Most group rides I have attended have set speed limits. This way you can join the group that most closely fits your own riding style.

Always maintain a safe following distance between you and other riders. Don't ride too close to the wheel in front of you. Leave enough space to react and brake safely.

While you are at it, try to ride as predictably as possible. Avoid sudden braking or swerving, since this can startle or affect riders behind you.

If you're at the front, use hand signals or call out to alert riders behind you to potholes, glass, or other dangers. Any sort of hazard that you see might be harder for someone in the back of the pack to spot.

When passing, pass on the left and communicate. If passing riders within your own group, announce "On your left" before you do so.

Ride single file on busy roads or narrow paths. On quiet roads or wide paths, riding two abreast might be acceptable if local rules permit it, and it doesn't impede others, but be ready to go single file quickly when needed.

This means riding just slightly ahead of the person next to you, which can feel competitive or uncomfortable. It's called half-wheeling, and it's considered rude behavior. Try to keep your handlebars roughly aligned with theirs if riding side-by-side.

By practicing these safe riding tips, you'll not only protect yourself but also enhance your enjoyment of every e-bike adventure. Remember, safety is an ongoing practice. Start slow, build your confidence, and never stop learning and observing. Happy and safe riding!

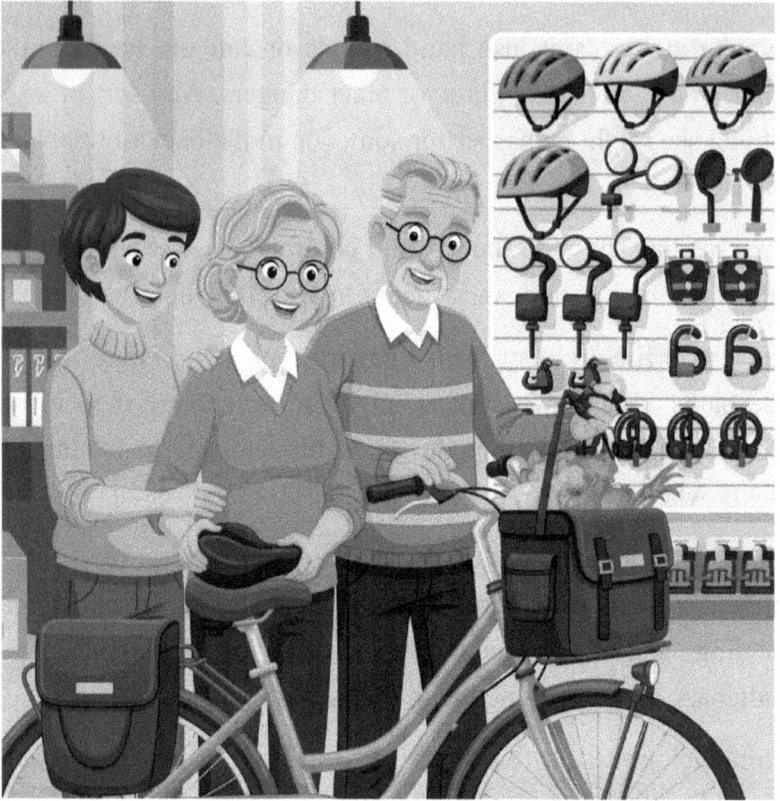

Chapter 12:
Must-have accessories for your new e-bike

NOTE: For a more detailed list of accessories, including my personal recommendations, be sure to check out the BONUS ACCESSORY APPENDIX at the end of the book.

You've chosen your perfect e-bike, and you're getting comfortable with riding it safely – fantastic! Now, I'd like to talk about a few key accessories that can significantly enhance your e-biking experience, making it safer, more comfortable, and more convenient. While some e-bikes come with a few basics, these additions are well worth considering. They will help you get the most out of your new ride. Think of them as the supporting cast that helps your star (your e-bike!) shine even brighter.

12.1. Lock

Protecting your investment. Your r-bike is a valuable item, both in terms of cost and the freedom it provides. Protecting it from theft is a top priority. A good quality lock is an absolute must-have.

There are several types of locks including:

U-Locks (or D-Locks)

These are generally considered one of the most secure types. They consist of a rigid U-shaped shackle and a crossbar. Look for one made from hardened steel.

Heavy-duty chain locks

These offer more flexibility in how you can lock your bike (e.g., around larger posts), but good ones can be quite heavy. Look for thick, hardened steel links and a robust lock mechanism.

Folding locks

Made of steel bars connected by rivets, these fold up compactly but can be less secure than a top-quality U-lock or chain.

Cable locks

While lightweight and convenient, cable locks are generally the least secure and are best used as a secondary deterrent (e.g., for securing your front wheel in addition to a U-lock on the frame and rear wheel) or for very short stops in low-risk areas.

Look for a high security rating. Many locks come with a security rating (e.g., Sold Secure in the UK, or ART in the Netherlands). Higher ratings mean better resistance to attack.

Consider where you'll carry the lock. Some U-locks come with frame mounts. Also remember some locks are very heavy. They might influence when and where you carry the lock.

Some locks use traditional keys, while others have combination dials. Keys get lost but then again, my memory isn't what it used to be!

Locking technique

Always lock your frame to a solid, immovable object (like a dedicated bike rack or sturdy pole). Remember to lock the frame first since that is the most valuable part of the e-bike.

If possible, also secure your rear wheel along with the frame. If you have a secondary cable lock, use it for the front wheel.

Make the lock as tight as possible, leaving little room for thieves to insert tools.

Never lock just the wheel, since a thief can remove the wheel and take the rest of the bike.

Investing $50-$150+ in a quality lock is a small price to pay for peace of mind. I have listed my favorites in the Appendix.

12.2. Panniers/baskets

Whether you're running errands, going for a picnic, or just need to carry an extra layer of clothing, having a way to transport items easily makes your e-bike much more practical.

Panniers are bags that attach to a cargo rack, usually mounted over the rear wheel. They offer significant carrying capacity and keep the weight low and stable. They are often waterproof or water-resistant. They're great for groceries, changes of clothes, or day-trip essentials.

There is one con to buying panniers. They require a rear rack to be installed (many e-bikes come with these, but not all.)

Baskets can be mounted on the front handlebars or on a rear rack. They make it easy to toss items in, good for quick trips, or carrying oddly shaped items. Front baskets keep items in view.

There is a con to using baskets. They can affect steering if a front basket is overloaded. Rear baskets are generally more stable.

You can also attach bags to the handlebars or to the seat.

These are typically much smaller bags used for essentials like your phone, wallet, keys, and a small snack. Handlebar bags are easily accessible, while saddle bags fit neatly under your seat.

When choosing bags, consider how much you typically need to carry. For many seniors, a set of easy-to-remove panniers or a sturdy rear basket offers excellent utility. If you just want to go as light as possible, these bags are a good choice.

12.3. Water bottle cage and bottle

Staying Hydrated. Hydration is important for everyone, especially when you're active. Having water easily accessible on your e-bike is a simple but crucial accessory. I live in the Southwest where there's high heat and low humidity. I also live at about 4,100 feet above sea level. I must hydrate every 20-30 minutes. It's not negotiable for me.

You can get a very inexpensive water bottle or cage to mount to your bike. Almost every e-bike sold has the capacity to accommodate this. It's a simple device that bolts onto pre-drilled holes on your e-bike frame. They're easy to install.

Look for a lightweight but sturdy design (aluminum or carbon fiber if you can afford it).

Make sure it holds a standard bicycle water bottle securely. Many water bottles are oversized and won't necessarily fit all cages.

Next, you'll need to choose a bottle that fits snugly in the cage. Insulated bottles can help keep your water cool on warmer days. Easy-to-open spouts are a plus when you need a quick sip. Make it a habit to take a water bottle with you on every ride, even shorter ones. I also prefer stainless steel because it doesn't pass forever chemicals with each drink.

12.4. Repair kit basics

Pump, spare tube, tire levers

While e-bikes are generally robust, a flat tire can happen to anyone. Being prepared with a few basic tools can turn a ride-ending frustration into a manageable inconvenience or at least allow you to get to a bike shop.

Consider a mini pump. This is a small, lightweight pump that attaches to your frame or fits in a bag. It takes effort to inflate a tire fully, but it's affordable and reliable.

Another option is a CO2 inflator. These use small cartridges of compressed CO2 to inflate a tire very quickly. Convenient but you need to carry spare cartridges. I personally find them too much trouble, but I also know people who love them.

Ensure the pump or inflator head is compatible with your tire valves—usually Presta or Schrader. Check your e-bike's tires. (Unless you are buying a racing bike that costs a whole lot of money you probably have Schrader valves.)

Carry a spare tube that is the correct size for your e-bike's tires. Your local bike shop can help you get the right one. If you carry your own, you'll save money, and you avoid the problem of showing up at a bike store that doesn't have what you need.

Carry tire levers. These small plastic levers (usually sold in sets of two or three) are essential for helping you remove the tire from the wheel rim to replace a punctured tube. Metal ones can damage your rim, so stick to plastic. These are dirt cheap so buy a bunch and have them on hand.

An optional but good backup is to carry a good patch kit. This is used for repairing a small hole in a tube if you don't have a spare or get a second flat. If you don't know how to fix the tire yourself, it still might make sense to carry one in case you run into someone who does know how to do it.

I also like to carry a compact multi-tool with various Allen keys (hex wrenches), and screwdrivers can be handy for minor adjustments on the go.

Store these items in a small saddlebag or pannier. Even if you don't feel confident doing the repair yourself, having the tools means a helpful passerby or a friend might be able to assist you. Knowing how to fix a flat is a great skill, and there are many helpful videos online, or your local bike shop might offer basic maintenance classes.

12.5. Comfort Upgrades

Saddle (seat) upgrades

Gel seat cover. An easy and relatively inexpensive way to add extra cushioning to your existing saddle.

Replacement saddle. If your stock saddle just isn't comfortable, consider a new one designed for comfort, perhaps wider with more padding or a central cutout for pressure relief. Bike shops often have "test" saddles you can try.

Ergonomic grips

These grips are shaped to provide better support for your palms and wrists, reducing pressure and numbness on longer rides.

Some have small "wings" or flared ends that distribute pressure more evenly.

They can make a noticeable difference in hand and wrist comfort.

Don't endure discomfort! Small changes here can transform your riding experience.

12.6. Phone mount

For navigation, entertainment or emergencies, your smartphone can be a valuable tool on your biking journey.

I use GPS apps for directions and exploring new routes. (My favorite is MapMyRide.) I also use the GPS on the phone to track my rides and to sync with my fitness apps.

In case of an emergency, you want to have your phone easily accessible in case you need to make a call.

I also use my phone to play my Spotify music over my earbuds.

A good phone mount attaches to your handlebars and securely holds your smartphone in view.

As you shop for a phone mount, be sure it has a secure grip. Ensure it holds your phone tightly, so it won't fall out on bumpy roads. You should also be able to easily insert and remove your phone.

The final two things to look for are adjustability—the ability to rotate the phone for portrait or landscape viewing—and weather resistance especially against rain.

Using a phone mount means you don't have to fumble in a pocket or bag to check your route or answer an important call, allowing you to keep your hands on the handlebars and your attention on riding.

Equipping your e-bike with these accessories will not only make your rides safer and more comfortable but also more practical and enjoyable. Choose the items that best suit your needs and riding style, and you'll be all set for many happy miles!

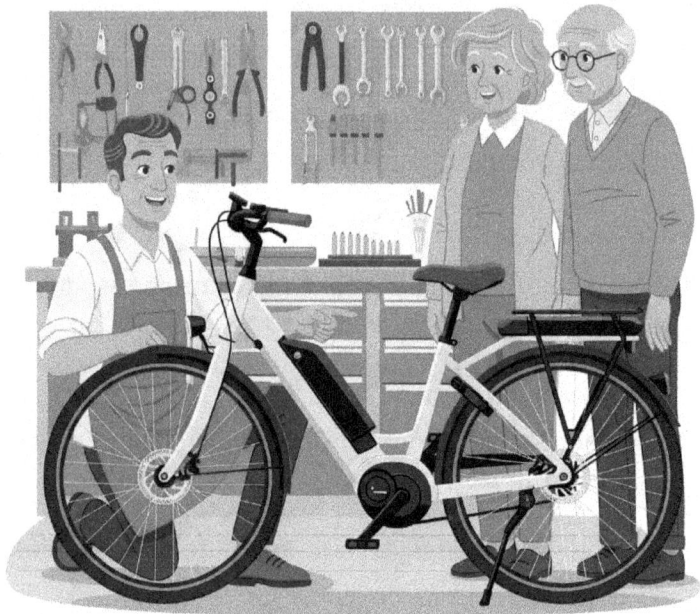

CHAPTER 13:
BASIC E-BIKE MAINTENANCE FOR SENIORS

Keeping your e-bike in good working order might sound intimidating, but it doesn't have to be! Just like tidying up your home or checking the oil in your car, a few simple, regular checks on your e-bike can make a huge difference. Basic maintenance ensures your rides are safer, smoother, and more enjoyable, and it helps your e-bike last longer.

You don't need to be a master mechanic. This chapter focuses on simple checks and tasks that most seniors can easily perform. Think of it as getting to know your bike a little better and building confidence in your ability to keep it rolling happily, whether you're heading to the market or just enjoying a spin around your neighborhood.

13.1. The ABC Quick Check (Plus 'e' for e-bike!)

This is the single most important habit you can develop. Before every single ride, take just two minutes to perform the "ABC Quick Check." It's a simple way to catch potential issues before they become problems on the road.

A is for Air. Are your tires properly inflated?

B is for Brakes. Do your brakes work correctly and feel responsive?

C is for Chain & Cranks. Is your chain looking okay, and are the pedals/cranks secure?

E is for Electrical. Is your battery charged and secure, and is the display working?

I will go into these with a little more detail. Making this quick check a pre-ride ritual provides immense peace of mind.

13.2. Tire pressure

Proper tire pressure is vital for several reasons. The first of which is safety. Underinflated tires can handle poorly, while overinflated ones offer less grip and a harsher ride.

Having correctly inflated tires also means your tires have less rolling resistance. That means your battery (and your legs) won't have to work as hard, extending your range.

(**Side note** – I ride a tire that is designed to be inflated to 30 PSI. I often run it at 23 PSI to give me a little more grip off-road and a little more comfort ON the road. But if I am going on a long ride, on paved surfaces and trying to stretch my battery, I will inflate the tires to 30 PSI to get the most distance I can from the charge.)

The right tire pressure helps absorb small bumps.

One of the biggest reasons not to underinflate your tires is a phenomenon known as "pinch flats." Also known as a "snake bite," a pinch flat is a type of bicycle tire puncture that occurs when the inner tube is squeezed between the tire and the rim, typically due to hitting a sharp edge like a curb or pothole with insufficient tire pressure. This impact forces the tire to compress, trapping and puncturing the tube, resulting in two small, parallel holes resembling a snake bite.

How to check your tire pressure

Look on the sidewall of your tire. You'll see a recommended pressure range—"Inflate to 40-65 PSI". You can use any standard tire gauge that you have around to check the pressure. The easiest way to check AND inflate is with a floor pump (also called a track pump). These are much easier to use than small hand pumps and almost always have a built-in pressure gauge.

Know your valve

There are two main types of tire valve. A Schrader (like the one you have on your car tires) and a Presta (thinner, with a small locking nut you unscrew before inflating). Most modern e-bikes sold in the USA have a Schrader valve. And the good news is that most pumps handle both.

Attach the pump head securely to the valve. Check the gauge. If it's low, pump until you reach a pressure within the recommended range. A good starting point is often the middle of the range. You can adjust slightly later based on comfort. Don't go above the maximum! Also be sure to regularly check the pressure. Aim to check your tire pressure at least once a week, and always before a long ride. My preference is to check before every ride. It only takes 30 seconds.

You can also buy a tire pump that uses compressed air to do the fill. This is what I use because it requires no physical effort from me, is fast and convenient. I list my favorite powered air compressor for e-bikes in the recommended accessory appendix.

One last thing. Do not be alarmed if you need to add some air occasionally. Tires naturally lose a little air over time.

13.3. Chain care: cleaning and lubrication

Your chain works hard! Keeping it clean and lubricated ensures smooth shifting, reduces wear on your expensive drivetrain components, and makes for a quieter ride. A little chain care goes a long way.

Take an old, clean rag and hold it around the lower part of the chain. Slowly turn the pedals backward, letting the chain run through the rag. This wipes off most of the surface dirt. For a deeper clean (only if very dirty), use a bike-specific degreaser and brushes, but be careful not to get degreaser on brake rotors or electrical parts. Often, a good wipe-down is enough. This is something you won't have to do very often if you own a modern day, e-bike. If you're constantly riding in sand, dirt, mud, water, etc., then you may need to clean the chain more often.

Some older bikes need more lubrication than the newer bikes. But as I said with chain cleaning, depending on where you ride, you might not need to do this all that often.

Get a bottle of bicycle-specific chain lube (ask your bike shop for a recommendation. A "dry lube" often works well in our climate). Do not use WD-40 or heavy oils! Slowly backpedal, applying one small drop of lube onto each roller (the little cylinders) of the chain. Keep backpedalling for 10-15 seconds to let the lube work its way in. Take a clean rag and wipe off all the excess lube. This is important! You only want lube inside the rollers, not all over the outside, where it just attracts dirt. Aim to lube your chain every few months, or more often if you ride in dusty conditions or hear it getting noisy.

13.4. Brake check: ensuring responsiveness

Your brakes are your most important safety feature.

Stand next to your bike and squeeze both brake levers. They should feel firm and engage before they hit the handlebar. They shouldn't feel "spongy" or "mushy."

Roll the bike forward and apply the front brake. Then roll it and apply the rear brake. Note how quickly or slowly the brakes work. This confirms they are engaging.

Look at your brake pads (the parts that squeeze the metal disc or rim). Can you see a good amount of pad material left? If they look very thin (less than 1-2mm) or you hear a grinding metal-on-metal sound, it's time for new pads.

Listen for excessive squealing or scraping sounds when braking. Some noise can happen (especially with disc brakes), but persistent, loud noises warrant a check. Unless you are experienced, do not attempt to adjust hydraulic disc brakes beyond simple checks. If they feel off, see a professional.

13.5. Tightening bolts

Things can occasionally loosen with vibration. You don't need to be a mechanic with a torque wrench (though that's the best way), but you can do simple checks.

Hold the front wheel between your knees and gently try to twist the handlebars. Is there any play? Does anything feel loose? Try to twist your saddle side-to-side. Does it move easily? It shouldn't. Ensure the seat post clamp is secure. If you have quick-release levers, make sure they are firmly closed. If you have thru-axles (solid bolts), ensure they feel snug. Gently wiggle any racks or fenders to ensure their mounting bolts aren't loose.

The key here is 'check.' If something feels obviously loose, tighten it gently or, better yet, ask your bike shop to check it and tighten it to the correct torque. Never over-tighten.

13.6. When to see a professional

I am very lucky because I have an excellent bike mechanic on call. He does mobile service, and if I need something, he usually shows up same day. It's important to know your limitations.

Knowing when to call in the experts is just as important as doing basic checks. Don't hesitate to visit a reputable local bike shop if:

- You hear persistent creaking, clicking, or grinding noises you can't identify.
- Your gears aren't shifting smoothly or reliably, even after chain care.
- Your brakes feel weak, spongy, or make loud noises.
- Your wheels wobble or don't spin freely.
- You experience any issues with the motor, battery (beyond charging), or display.
- You've had a fall or crash (even a minor one) It's crucial to have a pro check for hidden damage.
- You're unsure about any aspect of your bike's performance or safety.
- It's time for your regular tune-up (usually every 6 to 12 months, depending on how much you ride.

By incorporating these simple checks and care routines into your e-biking life, you'll not only protect your investment but also build confidence and ensure that every ride is as safe and enjoyable as possible. Now, let's get ready for Chapter 14, where I'll dive deeper into getting the most out of your battery.

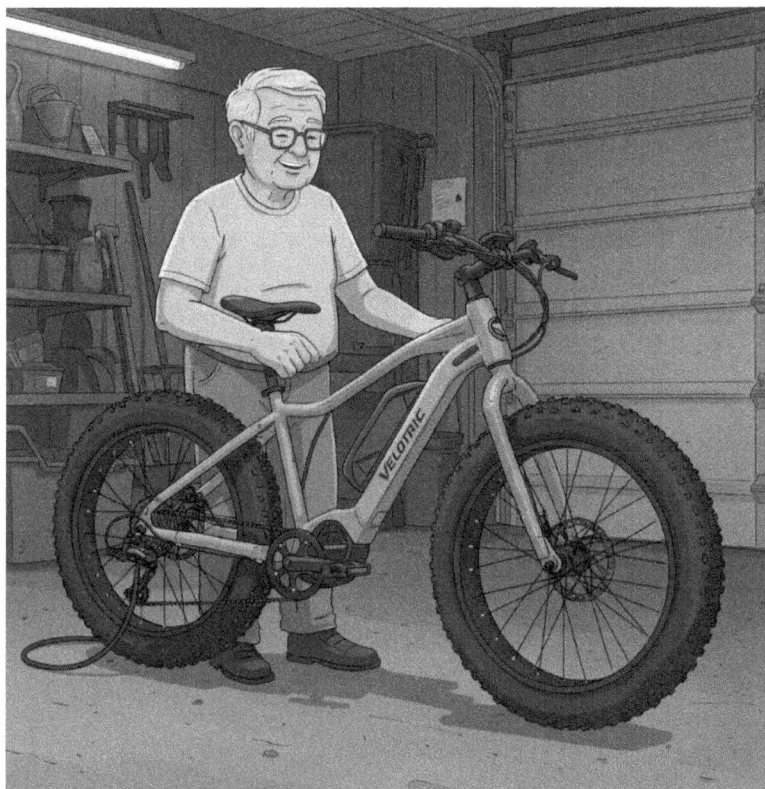

Chapter 14:
Maximizing your battery life and range

Your e-bike's battery is its heart. It's the source of that wonderful power that flattens hills, conquers distances, and brings the joy back to cycling. Understanding how to care for this vital component and how to get the most out of every charge is key to unlocking worry-free adventures, whether you're cruising along the river or planning a longer trip out into the far away hills.

One common concern for new e-bike riders is "range anxiety" – the fear of running out of power before reaching your destination. The good news is that with a little knowledge and a few good habits, you can significantly extend your battery's lifespan and maximize the distance you can travel on a single charge. I want to dive into how you can become the master of your e-bike's power source.

14.1. Charging best practices

Think of charging as refueling, but with a few simple rules to keep your battery healthy for years to come.

Use the right charger. This is non-negotiable. Always use the charger that came with your e-bike or an exact replacement specified by the manufacturer. Using the wrong charger can be ineffective at best and dangerous at worst, potentially damaging your battery or even posing a fire risk.

Avoid deep discharges. Lithium-ion batteries (the type used in most e-bikes) don't like being run completely empty. It's best to charge your battery before it gets critically low. Think about plugging it in when it reaches 20 to 30% capacity.

Don't worry about "overcharging." Modern, quality e-bike batteries have a built-in Battery Management System (BMS). This clever bit of technology automatically stops the charging process once the battery is full. So, while you can leave it plugged in overnight without much worry, it's generally a good practice to unplug it within a reasonable time after it's fully charged. This avoids any tiny, unnecessary "trickle" charges.

Know how often to re-charge. You don't need to charge your battery fully every single time you ride. In fact, frequent partial charges are perfectly fine for lithium-ion batteries. Many experts suggest that keeping your battery between 20% and 80% most of the time is ideal for longevity.

Aim for a full charge occasionally (perhaps once a month or so if you ride regularly) to help the BMS balance the cells.

After a long ride, especially on a hot day, your battery might be warm. It's a good idea to let it cool down to room temperature for 30 minutes to an hour before plugging in to charge. Similarly, let it cool a bit after charging before heading out again.

14.2. Battery storage tips

If you won't be riding your e-bike for a while (perhaps during the hottest part of summer or for an extended trip), how you store the battery matters.

Watch the temperatures. Batteries hate extremes. Never store your battery in direct sunlight, in a hot car, or in a freezing cold shed. The ideal storage temperature is generally between 50°F and 77°F (10°C to 25°C). If possible, remove the battery from the bike and store it indoors in a cool, dry place. A hot garage in July is not a good long-term storage spot.

Don't store your battery fully charged or fully empty for long periods. The sweet spot for long-term storage is typically between 40% and 60% charge.

If you're storing it for several months, check the charge level every month or two. If it drops below 30 to 40%, give it a short boost to bring it back into that ideal storage range. This prevents it from falling into a deep discharge state, which can permanently damage it.

14.3. Factors affecting range

Your e-bike might have an estimated range but think of that as a best-case scenario. The actual distance you can travel on a single charge depends heavily on several factors.

Your pedal assist system level impacts your battery life. This is the biggest one. Riding in "Turbo" or the highest assist level uses significantly more power than riding in "Eco" or the lowest level. Learning to use the lowest comfortable assist level for your situation is the single best way to maximize your range. Think of it like a car. Driving at 60 mph uses less fuel than driving at 90 mph.

Pay attention to your terrain. Riding on flat ground uses far less energy than climbing hills. Every incline demands more from your battery.

Rider weight and cargo. The more weight the bike must carry (rider + any groceries or gear), the more power it will use.

Tire pressure. Underinflated tires create more rolling resistance, making the motor work harder and reducing your range. Check your tire pressure regularly and keep it within the recommended range printed on the tire sidewall.

Wind. Riding into a strong headwind is like riding uphill. It dramatically increases resistance and eats up battery power.

Stopping and starting. City riding with frequent stops and starts uses more energy than maintaining a steady pace on an open trail. Temperature: While hot temperatures aren't great for storage, cold temperatures can temporarily reduce your battery's available capacity and range. By understanding these factors, you can make smarter choices while riding to extend your range and avoid getting caught short.

14.4. Replacing your battery

Like all rechargeable batteries, your e-bike battery won't last forever. Most e-bike batteries are rated for a certain number of charge cycles (typically 500 to 1,000 full cycles) or years of use. Eventually, you'll notice its capacity diminish. It won't hold as much charge or provide the range it used to. When that time comes, here's what to consider.

Signs it's time. A significant drop in range (e.g., a battery that used to give you 40 miles now only gives you 15) or a battery that won't hold a charge are clear signs.

Where to buy. The safest and most reliable option is to buy a replacement directly from your e-bike's manufacturer or an authorized dealer. This ensures compatibility and safety. While third-party options might exist and seem cheaper, they come with risks. They might not fit, perform well, or meet safety standards. If your bike has an extended warranty, a third-party battery might void that warranty.

Cost. E-bike batteries are a significant expense, often costing several hundred dollars or more. It's wise to factor this eventual cost into the long-term ownership of your e-bike.

Disposal. Never throw an old e-bike battery in the regular trash! They contain materials that require special handling and recycling. Your local bike shop or a local hazardous waste disposal facility can direct you on how to recycle it properly. Many shops will handle recycling when you purchase a new battery from them.

Your e-bike battery is a remarkable piece of technology. By treating it with a little care, understanding its needs, and being mindful of how you ride, you can ensure it serves you reliably for many miles and many years. Don't let range anxiety hold you back. Armed with this knowledge, you can confidently set out to enjoy all the fun, freedom, and fitness your e-bike has to offer.

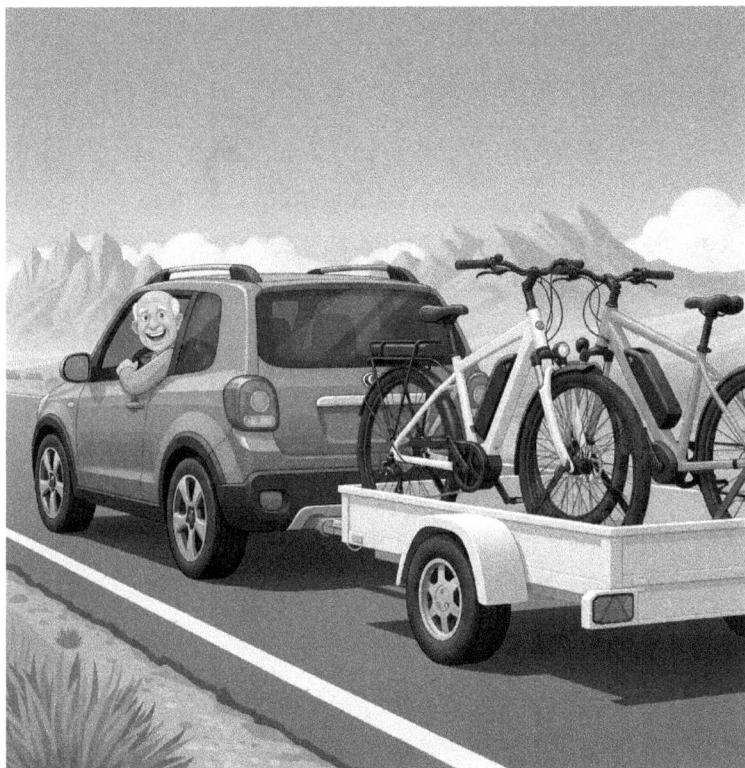

Chapter 15:
Storing and transporting
your e-bike

You've found your perfect e-bike, and you're enjoying the newfound freedom and fun it brings. That's fantastic! Now, let's talk about the practical side of ownership: where to keep your bike when you're not riding it, and how to take it with you when you want to explore trails or areas further afield from your home.

E-bikes are a bit heavier and bulkier than their traditional cousins. They're also a significant investment. Proper storage protects your bike from the elements and potential theft, while safe transport opens a whole new world of riding destinations. Planning these aspects will make your e-biking experience smoother and more enjoyable.

15.1. Home storage solutions

Finding the right spot at home involves balancing security, protection, and convenience.

For many, the garage is the go-to spot.

Pros: Generally secure, offers good protection from sun and rain.

Cons: Can get extremely hot in the summer (bad for batteries!), can become cluttered.

Tips: If your garage isn't insulated, always bring your battery inside, especially during hot summers and cooler winter nights (refer to Chapter 14 for battery storage tips).

Another option is a floor stand.

Simple, inexpensive, and require no lifting – just roll your bike in.

Another option is a wall mount. It can save floor space but be sure the mount is rated for the weight of your e-bike and is securely fastened to a wall stud. Lifting a 50-80 pound e-bike onto a hook can be challenging, so consider your physical abilities before choosing this option. Some clever pulley systems exist but ensure they are robust.

A note about secure storage.

Even in a locked garage, consider locking your e-bike to something solid. Same goes for sheds.

Apartment and indoor considerations

If you live in an apartment or prefer indoor storage, space is the main challenge.

Pros: Best protection from weather and theft, ideal temperature for battery storage.

Cons: Getting the bike inside (stairs, elevators), limited space.

Vertical Racks. Some stands store bikes vertically, taking up minimal floor space.

Look for designs that make it easy to pivot the bike up rather than requiring heavy lifting.

Wall hooks are another way to store your bike but use caution.

As with garages, ensure they can handle the weight, and you can safely lift the bike.

If space is a major concern, a folding e-bike might be an excellent choice, since they can often fit in a closet or corner. Use mats or trays to protect your floors from dirt and tire marks. Also consider your path. Can you easily navigate hallways and doorways? No matter where you store it, make sure it's convenient enough that getting your bike out isn't a major chore. You want to encourage riding, not create barriers!

15.2. Transporting your e-bike

Want to ride the trails near your local lake or mountain range? You'll likely need to transport your e-bike by car, truck, RV or trailer. This requires special consideration due to weight.

Most people start by getting a bike rack for their car. But be careful here. Most standard bicycle racks are NOT strong enough for e-bikes.

Attempting to use a standard rack can lead to rack failure, damage to your bike, damage to your car, and a serious road hazard. You must use a rack specifically designed for the weight and dimensions of e-bikes.

If you do get a rack, get a hitch-mounted rack. These are generally the best and safest option. They slide into your car's trailer hitch receiver (you'll need a hitch installed if you don't have one). The bike(s) sit on platforms and are secured with arms and straps.

They are good for e-bikes. They have high weight capacities (check the per-bike limit!), require less lifting than roof racks, and are very stable. Look for senior friendly features like ramps.

Many e-bike racks offer optional or integrated ramps. This is a game-changer, allowing you to simply roll your heavy e-bike up onto the rack instead of lifting it! Also opt for a rack with a low loading height. This makes lifting easier if a ramp isn't available.

Check how easy it is to secure the clamps and straps. Also know whether you have a 1.25" or 2" hitch receiver; most heavy-duty racks require a 2" hitch.

You can find trunk-mounted and roof-mounted racks, but I strongly advise you to steer clear of those because they make the process much more difficult.

Pro Tip: Remove your battery before transporting! Always take your e-bike battery off before putting your bike on a car rack because it reduces weight. Removing the battery can shave 7-10 lbs (or more!) off the weight you need to lift, carry or roll. This also protects the battery. It keeps your expensive battery safe inside the car from bumps, weather, and potential theft.

Removing the battery also lowers the center of gravity which makes the bike slightly easier to handle. If buying and installing a rack seems daunting, don't despair. Some bike shops offer rental racks or even transport services.

Taking a little time to set up a smart storage solution and invest in the right transport gear pays off handsomely. It protects your valuable e-bike, ensures your safety (and the safety of others on the road), and makes the whole process of getting out for a ride, whether from your front door or a distant trailhead, a simple pleasure.

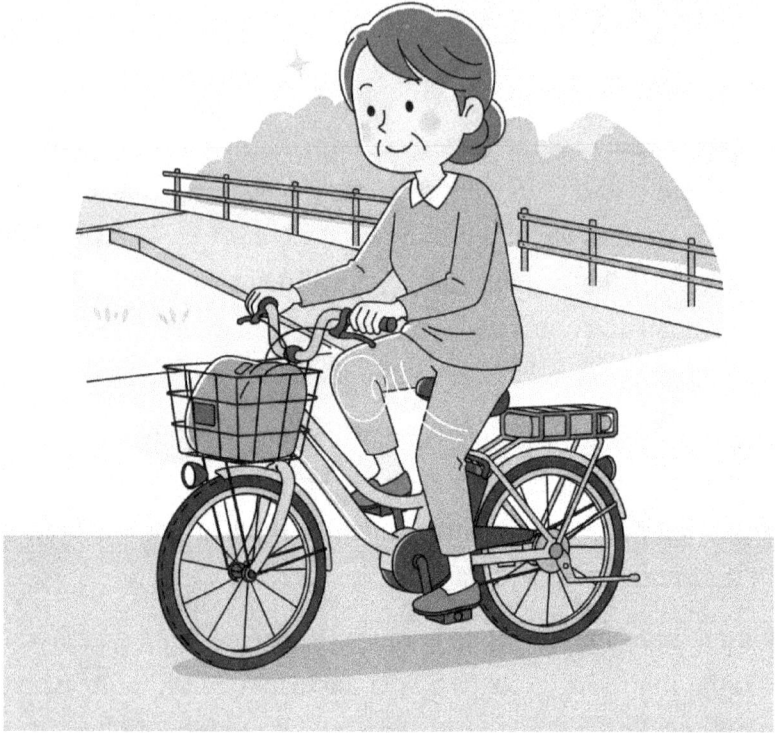

Conclusion:
Embrace the ride!

If you've stuck with me through the whole book, I want to say thank you and congratulations. As you've journeyed through these pages, you've likely transformed from someone perhaps cautiously curious about e-bikes into an informed, confident individual ready to embrace a new chapter of mobility, fun, and fitness.

I started by exploring why an e-bike is such a fantastic tool for seniors, demystified the technology, navigated the choices in bikes and accessories, and covered the essentials of safety, maintenance, and even how to get the most out of your battery. You've learned how to select a bike that fits your needs, how to store it, and even how to transport it for adventures further afield.

The journey from those first tentative questions to becoming a knowledgeable e-bike enthusiast is a significant one. You've equipped yourself not just with information, but with the potential for a richer, more active, and more independent lifestyle. The paths, trails, and quiet streets of your neighborhood, and indeed anywhere your heart desires, are now more accessible than ever.

Now, the most exciting part begins and that is the ride itself! Explore those routes you once thought too challenging. Revisit old favorite spots with a fresh perspective and less effort. Discover new cafes, parks, and scenic vistas. Feel the sun on your face and the gentle breeze as you pedal, knowing you have that reliable electric assist ready whenever you need it. This isn't just about exercise. It's about the sheer joy of movement, the thrill of discovery, and the incredible sense of freedom that your e-bike provides.

Remember, every ride is an opportunity. It's an opportunity to improve your health, to connect with your community, to reduce your carbon footprint, and simply to have a wonderful time. Don't be afraid to start small and gradually increase your distances as your confidence and fitness grow. There's no competition here, only personal enjoyment and well-being.

Perhaps you were hesitant at first, wondering if e-biking was truly for you. I hope this book has not only answered your questions but also ignited a spark of excitement. You have the knowledge, you have the tools, and now, hopefully, you have the motivation. Age is truly just a number when you have the right support – and your e-bike is a fantastic support system on wheels.

So, charge up that battery, put on your helmet, and embrace the ride. Your passport to fun, freedom, and fitness at any age is in your hands. The road ahead is open, and it's waiting for you.

Remember - It's never too late to roll!

Appendix 1:
Glossary of e-bike terms

Navigating the world of e-bikes can sometimes feel like learning a new language. This glossary will help you understand the common terms you'll encounter, making your journey to e-bike ownership and enjoyment smoother.

Ah (Ampere-hour or Amp-hour): A unit of electric charge. For e-bike batteries, it indicates the battery's capacity – how much energy it can store. A higher Ah rating generally means a longer potential range, assuming the same voltage. (See also Wh - Watt-hour).

Assist Levels: Settings on an e-bike that determine how much power the motor provides to help you pedal. Most e-bikes offer multiple levels, from low (eco mode, providing minimal assistance and maximizing range) to high (turbo or boost mode, providing maximum assistance for hills or speed, but using more battery).

Battery Management System (BMS): An electronic system built into the e-bike battery pack that monitors and manages its charging, discharging, temperature, and overall health. It protects the battery from overcharging, over-discharging, and overheating, prolonging its life and ensuring safety.

Bottom Bracket: The part of the bicycle frame where the crank arms (to which the pedals are attached) rotate. In mid-drive motors, the motor is often integrated around the bottom bracket.

Brakes (Disc): Most e-bikes use disc brakes, which offer superior stopping power, especially in wet conditions, compared to older rim brakes.

- Mechanical Disc Brakes: Use a cable to actuate the brake calipers.
- Hydraulic Disc Brakes: Use fluid in a sealed system to actuate the brake calipers, offering more power and better modulation (finer control). Highly recommended for e-bikes due to their weight and speed.

Cadence Sensor: A type of sensor used in some pedal-assist systems. It detects if the cranks are turning. If you are pedaling, regardless of how much effort you're putting in, the motor provides a set level of assistance based on your chosen assist level. (Compare with Torque Sensor).

Cassette: The stack of gears (cogs) on the rear wheel of the bicycle.

Chainrings: The toothed rings attached to the crank set at the front of the bike, which the chain engages with.

Charge Cycle: One complete discharge and recharge of a battery. For example, using half the battery's capacity and recharging it twice counts as one charge cycle. Battery lifespan is often rated in charge cycles (e.g., 500-1000 cycles).

Controller: The "brain" of the e-bike. It's an electronic component that takes input from the throttle (if equipped) and/or pedal-assist sensors and manages the flow of power from the battery to the motor.

Crank Arms (Cranks): The levers that connect the pedals to the bottom bracket and chainrings.

Derailleur: The mechanism that moves the chain from one gear to another on the cassette (rear derailleur) or chainrings (front derailleur, if present).

Direct-Drive Hub Motor: A type of hub motor that has no internal gearing. It's generally quieter but may offer less torque at low speeds compared to geared hub motors.

Drivetrain: All the components that transfer power from the rider (and motor) to the rear wheel. This includes the pedals, cranks, chainrings, chain, cassette, and derailleurs.

E-bike classes: In the United States, e-bikes are often categorized into three classes:

- Class 1: Pedal-assist only (no throttle), with assistance up to 20 mph.
- Class 2: Throttle-assisted (can be propelled without pedaling) and pedal-assist, with assistance up to 20 mph.
- Class 3: Pedal-assist only (no throttle), with assistance up to 28 mph. Often requires a speedometer.

Ergonomic Grips: Handlebar grips designed to provide better support for the hands and wrists, reducing pressure and fatigue. Often wider and flatter than traditional round grips.

Frame: The main structural component of the bicycle.

Step-Through Frame: A frame design with a very low or absent top tube, making it easier to mount and dismount. Highly popular with senior riders. Step-Over Frame (Diamond Frame): The traditional bicycle frame design with a higher top tube. Geared Hub Motor: A type of hub motor that uses internal gears. This allows the motor to be smaller and lighter while still providing good torque, especially for starting and climbing hills. They may produce a slight whirring sound.

Headset: The set of bearings that connects the fork to the frame and allows the handlebars and front wheel to turn.

Hub Motor: An electric motor located in the hub of either the front or rear wheel. (See also Direct-Drive Hub Motor and Geared Hub Motor).

Integrated Battery: A battery that is designed to fit smoothly into the e-bike's frame, often in the downtube, for a cleaner look and better weight distribution.

Kickstand: A retractable metal leg attached to the bike frame that allows it to remain upright when parked. Essential for heavier e-bikes.

Lithium-ion (Li-ion) Battery: The most common type of battery used in modern e-bikes. Known for their high energy density (more power in a smaller, lighter package) and longer lifespan compared to older battery technologies.

Mid-Drive Motor: An electric motor located at the center of the bike, near the bottom bracket, and integrated with the crank set. Mid-drive motors apply power directly to the drivetrain (chain), which can offer a more natural riding feel, better hill-climbing ability, and more efficient use of the bike's gears.

MIPS (Multi-directional Impact Protection System): A safety feature found in some bicycle helmets. It's a low-friction layer inside the helmet designed to allow a sliding motion of 10-15mm in all directions, reducing rotational motion transferred to the brain during an angled impact.

Modulation (Brake): The ability to finely control the amount of braking power applied. Good modulation allows for smooth, controlled stops rather than abrupt, jerky ones. Hydraulic disc brakes generally offer better modulation.

Panniers: Bags that attach to a rack (usually a rear rack) on either side of the wheel, used for carrying cargo like groceries, clothing, or gear.

Pedal Assist System (PAS): The system that provides power from the motor when you pedal. The amount of assistance is usually adjustable via different assist levels. (See also Cadence Sensor and Torque Sensor).

Quick Release (QR): A lever-operated mechanism used to easily attach or remove wheels or adjust the seat post height without tools. Less common on e-bike rear wheels with hub motors.

Range: The estimated distance an e-bike can travel on a single full battery charge. This is highly variable and depends on many factors, including battery capacity (Ah/Wh), assist level used, terrain, rider weight, tire pressure, and wind.

Regenerative Braking: A feature on some e-bikes (more common on direct-drive hub motors) where the motor acts as a generator when braking or coasting downhill, sending a small amount of charge back to the battery. The range extension is usually minimal but can help reduce brake wear.

Saddle: The bicycle seat. Comfort is key, especially for seniors. Gel saddles, wider saddles, and saddles with cutouts are popular options.

Suspension: Components designed to absorb shocks and vibrations from uneven surfaces, providing a smoother ride.

Front Suspension (Suspension Fork): Shock absorbers built into the front fork. Rear Suspension: Shock absorber(s) built into the rear of the frame (less common on city/commuter e-bikes, more common on e-mountain bikes).

Suspension Seat post: A seat post with a built-in spring or elastomer that absorbs bumps, adding comfort without the complexity of full frame suspension.

Throttle: A control (usually a twist grip or thumb lever on the handlebar) that allows the rider to engage the motor without pedaling. Common on Class 2 e-bikes. Some e-bikes have a "walk mode" throttle that provides minimal power to help push the bike.

Torque: A measure of rotational force. In e-bikes, motor torque (measured in Newton-meters, Nm) indicates how much power the motor can deliver, especially for starting from a stop or climbing hills. Higher torque generally means better acceleration and climbing ability.

Torque Sensor: A more sophisticated type of sensor used in some pedal-assist systems. It measures how hard the rider is pedaling. The motor then provides assistance proportional to the rider's effort – the harder you pedal, the more assistance you get. This often results in a more intuitive and natural-feeling ride compared to cadence sensor systems.

Tubeless Tires: Tires that do not require an inner tube. They use a special rim and sealant to create an airtight seal. They can often be run at lower pressures for better comfort and traction and are more resistant to pinch flats. Sealant can also automatically seal small punctures.

V (Volt): A unit of electric potential. e-bike batteries are typically 36V, 48V, or sometimes 52V. Higher voltage can mean more power delivery to the motor.

Walk Mode: A feature on many e-bikes that provides a low level of power to the motor when a button is pressed, making it easier to walk the bike alongside you, especially uphill or when it's loaded.

Wh (Watt-hour): A measure of total energy capacity in a battery. It's calculated by multiplying the battery's voltage (V) by its amp-hours (Ah). For example, a 36V, 10Ah battery has 360Wh. A higher Wh rating generally means a longer potential range. This is often the best single figure for comparing battery capacities.

APPENDIX 2:
ONLINE RESOURCES FOR 55+ E-BIKERS

The internet is a fantastic tool for learning more about e-bikes, connecting with fellow riders, and staying up to date on the latest news and regulations. Here is a curated list of online resources specifically chosen to be helpful for senior e-bike enthusiasts in the United States and Canada.

Online forums and communities

These are great places to ask questions, share experiences, and connect with other e-bike riders, including many seniors.

Electric Bike Review (EBR) Forums:

Website: https://electricbikereview.com/forums/

Description: Attached to one of the most comprehensive e-bike review sites, these forums are incredibly active and cover a vast range of topics. You can find discussions on specific brands and models, maintenance tips, and general e-biking chat. It's a great place to get real-world opinions, and many senior riders participate.

Endless Sphere DIY EV Forum (e-bike section):

Website: https://endless-sphere.com/sphere/

Description: While this forum leans towards the technical and do-it-yourself (DIY) aspects of electric vehicles, its e-bike section is a treasure trove of information. If you're technically inclined or want deep knowledge about motors and batteries, it's a valuable resource, though it can be a bit overwhelming for absolute beginners.

Cycling Without Age:

Website: https://cyclingwithoutage.org/

Description: While primarily an organization facilitating bike rides for less-mobile seniors using "trishaws," their website offers inspiration and resources. It highlights the social and well-being benefits of cycling and provides information on local chapters in both the U.S. and Canada, which can be a source of community connection.

E-Bike News, Reviews & Information Stay informed about new models, technology, and trends.

Electric Bike Review (EBR):

Website: *https://electricbikereview.com/*

Description: Arguably the most comprehensive e-bike review site online. It features detailed video and written reviews of hundreds of e-bikes, often categorizing them by use (like comfort or cruiser bikes, which are popular with seniors). The reviews are thorough, covering specs, ride feel, pros, and cons.

Electrek (See their e-bike section):

Website: https://electrek.co/guides/ebikes/

Description: A tech news site with a strong focus on electric transportation, including a dedicated e-bike section. It covers new model launches, industry news, and technological advancements. It's a good source for staying current.

Electric Bike Report

Website: https://electricbikereport.com/

Description: Offers a mix of in-depth reviews, news, guides (including buying guides and maintenance tips), and comparisons.

They often test bikes with a practical approach, which is useful for everyday riders.

Ebikes.org

Website: https://ebikes.org/

Description: A user-friendly site that aggregates reviews and allows you to compare different e-bike models. It provides rankings and guides to help you navigate the buying process.

Safety, education and advocacy

Learn about riding safely, understand regulations, and support cycling in your community.

League of American Bicyclists (LAB)

Website: https://bikeleague.org/

Description: A major U.S. advocacy group promoting safe and accessible cycling. Their website has extensive resources on bike safety (including tips for older adults), educational programs (Smart Cycling), bike laws by state, and information on e-bikes.

PeopleForBikes

Website: https://www.peopleforbikes.org/

Description: This U.S.-based group advocates for better biking infrastructure and policies. Their site includes information on e-bike regulations across different states, statistics, and resources for riders.

Parachute (Canada)

Website: https://parachute.ca/en/injury-topic/cycling/

Description: Canada's national charity dedicated to injury prevention. Their cycling section provides valuable safety tips, information on helmet laws, and resources relevant to Canadian cyclists.

Canadian Automobile Association (CAA) / American Automobile Association (AAA)

Websites: https://www.caa.ca/driving-safely/cycling/ (Canada) & https://exchange.aaa.com/safety/bicycle-safety/ (USA)

Description: Both organizations offer resources on road sharing, bicycle safety rules, and sometimes specific information on e-bikes, often with a focus on interaction with motor vehicles.

CyclingSavvy

Website: https://cyclingsavvy.org/ebike-safety-resources/

Description: An organization focused on teaching cyclists how to ride safely and confidently in various traffic situations. They have a dedicated section with e-bike safety resources and online courses.

Appendix 3:
My preferred accessory list

This is a list of my favorite accessories that I personally use. In each case, I paid full price for the item, and I have no relationship with any of the manufacturers. I am an Amazon affiliate and if you use my links, I get a very small commission on each item. It doesn't impact the price you pay.

DISCLAIMER: I am not saying YOU should buy these accessories - only that I did buy them and kept them and use them. I do endorse them and am happy with them or I wouldn't have kept them. I offer this list simply as a look at my personal choices. Hopefully it will help you find what's best for you.

Also note the prices listed reflect what I paid. By the time you read this, the prices may have changed.

Seat

I am 6.1/2" tall a big guy, and I need a big seat. I probably could have gotten by with the stock seat, but I have one of these on my other e-bike and have grown to really like it, so I swapped seats and replaced it with:

Wuvop Oversized Peloton Bike Seat (https://amzn.to/3ZzBIBz)

$33.95

Grips

The Nomad II comes with very good grips, but I wanted to add bar-end mirrors and these grips come equipped with a removable end cap that makes it easier to install the mirror.

My Budget Pick:

ROCKBROS Bike Handle Grips (https://amzn.to/3HJ5TAo)

$19.99

My Pro Pick:

Ergon GP1 Mountain Bike Grips (https://amzn.to/4onH2Ti)

$36.95

Camera mount

I occasionally use my GoPro Hero 11 to make videos while riding. I tested a dozen handlebar mounts, and this one is inexpensive and works very well.

Sametop Bike Pole Mount (https://amzn.to/45cd6AO)

$18.99

Side mirrors

The Nomad doesn't come with mirrors. I ordered five different sets I didn't like (including the one Velotric sells) and ended up picking some inexpensive bar-end mirrors that were recommended to me by more than a dozen trusted sources. They work great.

Mirrycle MTB Bar End Mountain Bicycle Mirror (https://amzn.to/4kRDbf9)

$15.26 x2

Pedals

The Nomad - like most bikes in its price category comes with cheap pedals. There's nothing wrong with them, but I wanted a slightly wider platform, and I'm happy I made the change.

BUCKLOS Mountain Bike Pedals MTB Pedals Flat (https://amzn.to/4jT4aG2)

$21.36

Bottle cage

I want to stay hydrated when I ride, and the Nomad has built in screws and a place for a bottle holder. This is the one I use.

HUALONG Ultra Light Full Carbon Fiber Water Bottle Cage (https://amzn.to/44aPYlY)

$22.90

Water bottle

Again - as part of my hydration strategy. I wanted something that wouldn't leave me full of forever chemicals, so I spent money on a really good bottle from a brand highly recommended by cyclists.

CamelBak Podium Steel Insulated Stainless Steel Bike Water Bottle (https://amzn.to/3G0fkux)

$44.00

Bright auxiliary front/rear LED lights

Most car/bike accidents happen because the car driver just isn't looking for bikes. Having an auxiliary set of blinking LEDS is crucial for visibility, especially in low-light conditions.

I've gone through five different sets of these types of lights, looking for the best balance of performance and price. I had some issues with other models I like needing to be recharged too often so I am now using these.

Prasky LED Bike Lights (https://amzn.to/3J5Z0cQ)

$19.94

Bright Rear Warning Light/Radar

Blinking light and rearview radar with taillight provides awareness of vehicles approaching from behind up to 153 yards (140 meters) away

Garmin Varia RTL515 (https://amzn.to/4eXHS4Q)

$199.99

High-visibility vest or clothing

Brightly colored or reflective vests, jackets, or even arm/leg bands significantly increase a rider's visibility to motorists and pedestrians. I look like a member of the Village People when I ride, but I AM visible.

Salzmann Mesh Multi-Pocket Working Vest - Reflective Vest (https://amzn.to/3SSQL5O)

$14.90

Men's padded mountain bike shorts

I can ride 15-20% further wearing these shorts compared to not wearing them so if I want distance/time on the bike, these are my go-to.

https://amzn.to/4lN9HzC

$29.99

High visibility rain jacket

It rarely rains where I live and is usually warm but for the few times when it's needed, I want a lightweight, hi-vis jacket to wear. This is my favorite.

Men's Cycling Rain Jacket Waterproof Running Bike Windbreaker

https://amzn.to/3GtthBC

$49.99

Riding gloves

FULL-FINGER - I like to wear gloves to protect my hands from road debris, to protect my hands if I fall, and to help reduce vibration from the handlebars. This pair from GripGrab is favored by many serious cyclists.

GripGrab SuperGel XC Padded Full Finger Summer Cycling Gloves

GripGrab - https://amzn.to/3TuvnUB

$44.99

HALF-FINGER - For me - the Castelli Arenberg Gel 2 gloves are essential for comfort. They are a top-tier contender. What sets these gloves apart for the e-bike enthusiast is the exceptional vibration damping provided by the Castelli Damping System (CDS), which strategically places gel padding to protect the median nerve and reduce the hand numbness that can creep in after miles on the road.

Castelli Arenberg Gel 2 - https://amzn.to/4kvqCFu

$49.99

Helmet with MIPS

For me, a good quality, properly fitting helmet is a must. Technologies like MIPS (Multi-directional Impact Protection System) can offer additional protection. I also have a large head, and the Giro brand is one of the few that make a helmet which fits me.

Giro Fixture MIPS Adult Mountain Cycling Helmet (https://amzn.to/3SP7gzJ)

$62.45

Security

Good locks will protect your investment. Nothing you or I do will keep your bike and belongings safe from a determined thief. But you can slow them down and discourage random theft attempts with a good lock OR two OR three...

- HELMET - LOCK the one I picked is designed for motorcyclists but works well for e-bikers too.
  ROCKBROS Motorcycle Helmet Lock (https://amzn.to/4e2G4Y5)
  $9.99
- Bike lock #1
  RBRL Bicycle Lock (https://amzn.to/3TpZgoY)
  $55.99
- Bike lock #2
  HIPLOK Z Lok Single Zip Combo Lock (https://amzn.to/43S7YB6)
  $45.22

Tire puncture protection

I live in New Mexico where we have a ton of goat heads - they are nasty little stickers that took down my tires nearly every time I rode - even on paved paths. I tried three different brands of sealant before I settled on this one - haven't had a flat since.

Flat Out QuickStrike Tire Sealant Off-Road Formula (https://amzn.to/45WjVbH)

$23.99

Tire pressure gauge

I keep this gauge in my garage to use to test my tires before I ride. It's too big to carry with me but I only need it as part of my safety check. It's longer than most and is easy on my back since I do not have to stay bent over for too long.

GODESON Tire Pressure Gauge (https://amzn.to/3ZZWCtO)

$11.99

Portable air pump/compressor:

While puncture-resistant tires help, it's always good to be prepared. A relatively small, easy-to-use pump and a simple patch kit can be lifesavers. I can put this unit in my rear trunk bag. There are smaller ones, but this is the one my bike mechanic uses and recommends so it was good enough for me. Works fast, easy and reliably.

Ryobi RPI18-0 High Pressure Compressor (https://amzn.to/3TnFcU6)

$39.00

Battery for Ryobi Compressor

Ryobi One+ 18v Lithium Ion 2.0ah Battery and Charger Kit (https://amzn.to/4002vao)

$55.90

Bike Trunk Bag

Provides convenient storage for groceries, personal items, or a jacket. Baskets are easy to access, while panniers and trunk bags offer more secure and water-resistant storage. I prefer this to paniers.

Ibera MIK Commuter Bag (https://amzn.to/44folJs) (NOTE - Need a MIK system for this to work. It works for me because my bike comes with a MIK system.)

$124.99

Phone Mount

Having a cell phone mount allows for easy viewing of navigation apps or tracking ride stats. I originally used the mount from Velotric - I used to believe the manufacturer's mount is always the safe choice, but recently my phone came flying out of the Velotric phone holder when I hit a bump, so I went searching for a new mount. Then I tried the Quad Lock Out Front Pro. It's VERY expensive since you really need a new phone case. It was a bear to install, and I never got it to fit my Velotric handlebars the way I wanted so I sent it back and opted for an inexpensive unit called:

Lamicall Motorcycle Bike Phone Mount - https://amzn.to/4o8q1wt

$17.99

Bell

I tried four different bells. Some of them very expensive and most very inexpensive. The one I liked best was inexpensive. Easy to mount and plenty loud.

ROCKBROS Bike Bell Classic Bicycle Bell Mountain - https://amzn.to/3GLPWJC

$14.99

CONCLUSION

I tend to customize everything I buy. Many of you reading this will never need any of these accessories (if you already have a helmet.) There's no need to feel pressure to buy ANYTHING. But if you DO want to accessorize your e-bike, I hope you find this list helpful. These items have improved my e-biking experience.

APPENDIX 4:
PRE-RIDE CHECKLIST

This is a detailed look at my pre-ride checklist. It is e-bike specific. This entire list takes just a couple of minutes and can prevent common issues.

A - Air

[ ] Check tire pressure using a gauge. Inflate to the recommended PSI (pounds per square inch) printed on the tire sidewall. Proper pressure prevents flats, improves range, and ensures good handling.

B - Brakes

[ ] Squeeze brake levers. They should feel firm, not spongy, and stop the wheels effectively.

[ ] Visually inspect brake pads for wear.

[ ] Listen for any scraping or squealing sounds.

C - Chain and cranks

[ ] Look at the chain. Is it relatively clean and lightly lubricated? (Don't over-lube).

[ ] Check cranks (pedal arms) to ensure they are tight and not wobbly.

E - Electrical system (e-bike specifics)

[ ] Check battery charge level. Is it sufficient for your planned ride?

[ ] Ensure battery is securely mounted.

[ ] Turn on the display. Are all indicators working correctly?

[ ] Test lights (if equipped).

Quick release/thru-axles

[ ] Ensure wheels are securely attached. Check quick-release levers or thru-axles for tightness.

Helmet check

[ ] Inspect your helmet for any cracks or damage. Ensure straps are adjusted correctly.

II. Weekly (or every five to 10 rides)

Clean your e-bike

[ ] Wipe down the frame, fork, and components with a damp cloth. Avoid spraying water directly onto electrical components, battery housing, or motor.

[ ] Clean the chain with a rag and chain cleaner/degreaser if it's very dirty.

Lubricate chain

[ ] Apply a quality bicycle chain lubricant sparingly to the chain rollers while backpedaling.

[ ] Wipe off excess lubricant with a clean rag. Too much lube attracts dirt.

Inspect tires more closely

[ ] Check for embedded glass, thorns, or cuts in the tire tread and sidewalls.

[ ] Check for signs of excessive wear.

[ ] Check bolts and fasteners

[ ] Visually inspect key bolts (handlebars, stem, seatpost, racks, fenders) to ensure they appear tight. If you have a torque wrench and

know the specs, you can check them properly. Otherwise, if something feels loose, have a mechanic check it.

Check brake functionality

[ ] Test brakes again. Ensure smooth operation and good stopping power.

III. Monthly (or every 20-30 rides)

[ ] Deeper drivetrain clean

[ ] Thoroughly clean the chain, cassette (rear gears), and chainrings using brushes and a bike-specific degreaser.

[ ] Re-lubricate the chain after cleaning.

Inspect brake pads and rotors

[ ] Check brake pads for wear. Most have wear indicators. Replace if worn down.

[ ] Inspect disc brake rotors for any warping or deep scoring. Clean with isopropyl alcohol if they seem contaminated.

Check cables and housing

[ ] Inspect brake and gear cables (if mechanical) for fraying, rust, or kinks.

[ ] Check cable housing for cracks or damage.

Check wheel trueness

[ ] Spin wheels and look for any significant side-to-side wobble. Minor adjustments may be needed by a mechanic if wobbles are present.

Check headset

[ ] Apply the front brake and gently rock the bike back and forth. Feel for any looseness or knocking in the headset (where the fork meets the frame). If loose, it needs adjustment by a mechanic.

Check pedal tightness

[ ] Ensure pedals are securely tightened into the crank arms.

Inspect electrical connections (e-bike specific)

[ ] Visually inspect any visible electrical connectors for corrosion or damage. Ensure they are securely connected. Do not unplug or tamper with connections unless you are confident and following manufacturer instructions.

IV. Every six months (or every 500-750 miles)

Professional tune-up recommended

Take your e-bike to a qualified e-bike mechanic for a comprehensive tune-up. This typically includes:

- Brake adjustments and pad replacement if needed
- Gear indexing and derailleur adjustments
- Wheel truing and spoke tension check
- Checking and tightening all bolts to correct torque specifications
- Headset and bottom bracket check/adjustment
- Drivetrain wear inspection (chain, cassette, chainrings)
- Software updates for motor/battery system (if applicable and available)
- Overall safety inspection.

Check chain wear

[ ] Use a chain wear indicator tool to check for chain stretch. Replace the chain if it's worn to prevent excessive wear on more expensive cassette and chainrings.

Inspect and clean battery terminals (e-bike specific)

[ ] With the battery removed and power off, gently inspect the battery terminals on both the battery and the bike frame for any dirt or corrosion. Clean carefully with a dry cloth or a pencil eraser if needed. Ensure they are dry before reinstalling the battery.

V. **Annually (or Every 1000-1500 Miles)**

[Comprehensive professional service (strongly recommended)

- This builds on the six-month tune-up and may include:
- Overhaul or replacement of bearings (hubs, headset, bottom bracket) if needed.
- Replacement of cables and housing.
- Hydraulic brake fluid bleed/replacement if needed.
- Suspension fork service (if equipped).
- Thorough inspection of all components for wear and tear.

Battery health check (e-bike specific)

[ ] Some bike shops with e-bike diagnostic tools can perform a battery health check to assess its capacity and overall condition.

VI. **As needed**

After riding in wet or muddy conditions

[ ] Clean your e-bike as soon as possible to prevent rust and grime buildup. Pay extra attention to the drivetrain.

[ ] Re-lubricate the chain.

If you hear unusual noises

[ ] Investigate squeaks, creaks, or grinding sounds promptly. They often indicate a problem that needs attention.

After a brash or impact

[ ] Thoroughly inspect the frame, fork, wheels, and all components for damage before riding again. If in doubt, have a mechanic inspect it.

Tire Replacement

[ ] Replace tires when the tread is worn down, if there are significant cuts or damage to the sidewalls, or if you experience frequent flats.

By following this maintenance schedule, you'll not only extend the life of your e-bike and its components but also ensure a safer and more enjoyable riding experience every time you head out. Happy E-biking!

Appendix 5: Detailed pre-purchase checklist

Are you ready to buy your e-bike?

Buying an e-bike is an exciting step towards new adventures, improved fitness, and greater freedom. This checklist is designed to help you think through the key considerations before making your purchase, ensuring you choose an e-bike that perfectly suits your needs and preferences. Take your time, do your research, and get ready to embrace the ride!

Section 1: Understanding your needs and goals

Primary Use: What will you mainly use your e-bike for?

[ ] Leisurely rides and recreation

[ ] Fitness and exercise

[ ] Running errands and local commuting

[ ] Exploring trails (paved, light gravel)

[ ] Longer distance touring

Riding Terrain

Where will you be riding most often?

[ ] Mostly flat surfaces (e.g., Las Cruces River trails)

[ ] Areas with moderate hills

[ ] Steep hills that require significant assistance

[ ] Paved paths and city streets

[ ] Light gravel or unpaved trails

[ ] Desired range: How far do you typically want to ride on a single charge?

[ ] Short trips (under 20 miles)

[ ] Medium trips (20-40 miles)

[ ] Longer trips (over 40 miles)

Physical considerations

[ ] Do you have any mobility issues that would make mounting/dismounting difficult? (Consider step-through frames)

[ ] Do you experience back, wrist, or neck discomfort? (Consider upright riding posture, ergonomic grips, suspension)

[ ] Are you comfortable with the weight of an e-bike for handling and potential lifting?

Budget

What is your comfortable budget range for the e-bike and essential accessories?

[ ] E-bike: $_____ to $_____

[ ] Accessories (helmet, lock, lights, etc.): $_____

Section 2: Key e-bike features to consider

Frame style

[ ] Step-through (easier to mount/dismount)

[ ] Step-over (traditional diamond frame)

Motor type and power

[ ] Mid-drive motor (often better for hills and natural feel)

[ ] Hub motor (can be front or rear, often more budget-friendly)

[ ] Is the motor torque (Nm) sufficient for your expected terrain?

Battery

[ ] Is the battery capacity (Wh or Ah/V) adequate for your desired range?

[ ] Is the battery easily removable for charging indoors?

[ ] Integrated vs. External battery (aesthetic and protection preference)

[ ] **E-bike class (Check your local community regulations)**

[ ] Class 1 (Pedal-assist up to 20 mph)

[ ] Class 2 (Throttle + Pedal-assist up to 20 mph)

[ ] Class 3 (Pedal-assist up to 28 mph)

Brakes

[ ] Hydraulic disc brakes (highly recommended for stopping power and control)

[ ] Mechanical disc brakes

Suspension

[ ] Front suspension fork (for comfort on bumps)

[ ] Suspension Seatpost (adds significant comfort)

[ ] Full Suspension (less common for typical senior use, more for off-road)

Tires

[ ] Wider tires for stability and comfort?

[ ] Puncture-resistant tires or liners?

Weight of e-bike

[ ] Are you comfortable with the overall weight for maneuvering and potential lifting (e.g., onto a rack, over a curb)?

Sensor type (pedal assist)

[ ] Torque sensor (more intuitive, assistance based on pedaling effort)

[ ] Cadence sensor (assistance based on cranks turning)

Gears (drivetrain)

[ ] Sufficient range of gears for your terrain?

[ ] Easy-to-use shifters?

Display and controls

[ ] Is the display easy to read (speed, battery level, assist level)?

[ ] Are the controls intuitive and easy to reach?

Section 3: Research and shopping process

Brands and models

[ ] Have you researched different e-bike brands and specific models that seem suitable?

[ ] Reviews – Have you read reviews from other owners, particularly seniors if possible?

[ ] **Local bike shops**

[ ] Visited reputable local bike shops in the Las Cruces area?

[ ] Discussed your needs with knowledgeable staff?

[ ] Inquired about after-sales service and support?

Online retailers

[ ] If considering online, have you researched assembly requirements?

[ ] Understood how warranty and service are handled for online purchases?

Warranty

[ ] Do you understand the warranty coverage for the frame, motor, battery, and other components?

Section 4: The all-important test ride

Multiple models

[ ] Have you test-ridden at least two to three different e-bikes?

Comfort check

[ ] Does the saddle feel comfortable?

[ ] Are the handlebar grips comfortable?

[ ] Is the riding posture comfortable for your back, neck, and wrists?

[ ] Can you easily reach the ground when stopped (or adjust the seat to do so)?

Assist levels

Did you try all the pedal-assist levels? Do they feel smooth and provide the right amount of support?

Brakes

[ ] Do the brakes feel powerful and easy to control?

[ ] Handling

Do you feel confident and stable handling the bike, including starting, stopping, and turning?

Motor noise

[ ] Is the motor noise level acceptable to you?

[ ] Throttle (if Class 2): If it has a throttle, did you test its responsiveness?

Section 5: Essential accessories and gear

Helmet

[ ] Have you selected a comfortable, well-fitting helmet (MIPS technology recommended)?

Lock

[ ] Do you have a high-quality lock (U-lock or heavy-duty chain) to secure your investment?

[ ] Lights – Does the e-bike have integrated lights? If not, have you chosen bright front and rear lights?

Storage/Cargo

[ ] Rack for carrying items?

[ ] Basket or Panniers?

Mirror

For visibility of traffic behind you?

[ ] Bell or horn

[ ] To alert pedestrians and other cyclists?

Other comfort Items

[ ] Upgraded saddle or seat cover?

[ ] Ergonomic grips?

[ ] Suspension seatpost (if not included)?

[ ] Basic repair kit: (patch kit, tire levers, mini pump)

Section 6: Storage and transportation plans

Home storage

[ ] Do you have a secure, dry place to store your e-bike at home?

[ ] Is the storage area protected from extreme temperatures (especially for the battery)?

[ ] Is there convenient access to an outlet for charging?

[ ] Transportation (if needed):

[ ] If you plan to transport your e-bike by car, have you researched e-bike specific car racks (hitch-mounted platform racks with ramps are often best)?

[ ] Is your vehicle equipped with the necessary hitch?

Section 7: Safety and legal awareness

Local Laws

 Are you familiar with the e-bike laws and regulations in your city and state? (e.g., where Class 1, 2, or 3 e-bikes are permitted)?

Safe riding practices

[ ] Have you reviewed safe cycling practices?

Insurance

[ ] Have you considered if your homeowner's or renter's insurance covers your e-bike, or if you need separate e-bike insurance?

Section 8: Post-purchase considerations

Basic maintenance

[ ] Do you understand the basic maintenance your e-bike will require (e.g., tire pressure, chain lubrication, cleaning)?

Service provider

[ ] Do you know where you will take your e-bike for regular servicing or repairs? (Often the shop where you purchased it).

If you can confidently check off most of the items on this list, you are well on your way to making a fantastic e-bike purchase. Congratulations on taking this step towards enhanced mobility and enjoyment!

MY STORY

My name is Scott and I'm passionate about e-bikes and even more passionate about convincing others 55 and older to give them a try. I've personally found so much joy and freedom thanks to e-biking.

My e-bike journey and experience

My first bike was a 1963 Schwinn Stingray, but it was unfortunately stolen a year after my uncle gave it to me. After that, any bikes I had were just hand-me-down "junkers" that no other kid wanted.

As I grew up, I occasionally rode a bicycle.

When I lived in San Francisco's SOMA neighborhood, I commuted to my office on Potrero Hill on my bike. But as life sped by and I travelled a lot for work, I rarely rode.

That all changed in 2014. Out of shape and semi-retired, I decided to buy my first e-bike. I chose a Pedego Interceptor because there was a dealer nearby. I'd never ridden an e-bike, or any bike, for 13 miles, but on that day, I rode my new e-bike from the dealership to my home and was completely hooked.

In 2017, I upgraded to the Platinum edition of the Interceptor. This was a big improvement, and I found myself riding every day. I lived near a path designed for walkers and riders, which really helped me stay on the bike. That year, I lost 40 pounds, got off my blood pressure medication, and was healthier than I'd been in years.

Then, I took a job that paid well but demanded 80 hours a week. I was constantly on airplanes or behind a computer, and I didn't ride for many months. I gained the weight back (and then some), went back on meds, and became very sick.

After I left that job, I was so unsteady that I couldn't even lift my leg over the crossbar of the Interceptor, so I bought a newer, step-through version. My health was still poor, limiting how much I could ride, but at least I was back on a bike.

A new chapter in New Mexico

Fast forward to 2024, and my health was still in decline. I was still living in the Seattle area, and the constant rain and cold left me unmotivated. I sold my step-through and started thinking about making a change.

On the advice of my doctor, I bought a trike – the Pedego Fat Tire Trike – and moved to sunny, warm New Mexico. I now live in Las Cruces, an area surrounded by bike trails and paths, with 13 parks within 2.2 miles of my new home.

I started riding every day again and eventually regained my balance. I even added a second e-bike to my stable: a Velotric Nomad 2.

Where has all this led? I'm happier than I've been in 20 years. I get to feel the wind in my face and the warmth of the sun on my skin. I get to see, hear, and even smell the area around me. I wave to my neighbors (who are all very curious about my e-bikes, especially the trike), and I get to live a life that doesn't involve sitting in front of a computer.

I've lost 95 pounds (some of that was due to diet changes, none from weight loss drugs), and at 70 years old, with a heart condition and severe osteoarthritis, I've even stumped my doctors, who don't understand why I'm doing so well.

And that right there, folks, is the reason I wrote this book. My message is if I can do it, anyone can do it. I'm here to motivate you to take that leap of faith so you can feel better too.

I volunteer my time and resources at a local bicycle charity and spend the rest of my time riding or hosting the "Senior-Biker Podcast" and newsletter/website (seniorebiker.substack.com). It's all part of my ongoing commitment to building a community and resource hub for senior e-bike riders.

I'm excited to be more mobile than ever and hope the information in this book motivates others my age to give e-biking a try.

REMEMBER, IT'S NEVER TOO LATE TO ROLL.

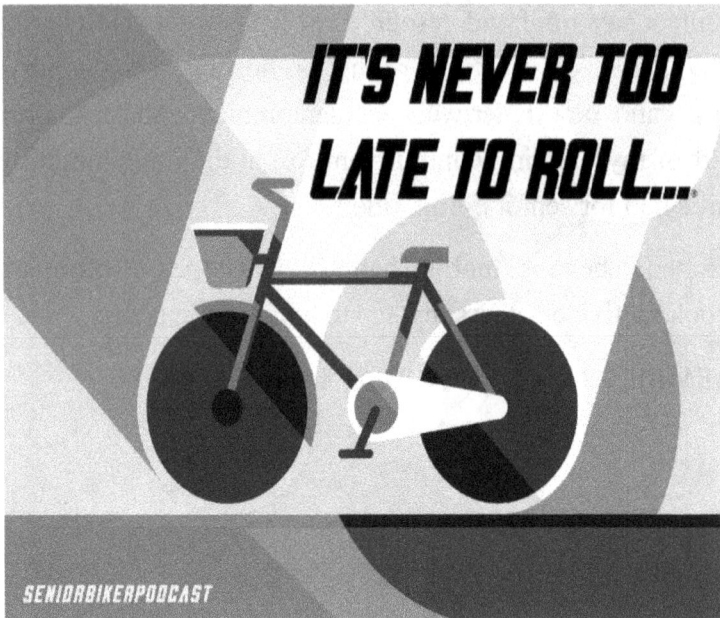

Want to learn more?

Check out the Senior E-biker Podcast. The first and third Tuesday of each month, I publish a free podcast (available wherever you listen to all your favorite shows) full of useful information, news, tips, tricks and reviews about E-biking with the 55+ rider in mind.

You can visit the Senior E-biker Podcast home page at:

https://senior-ebiker.transistor.fm

I publish a free newsletter on Substack. You do not have to pay to read my posts. The newsletter can also be e-mailed to you if you sign up. You can find it at: https://seniorebiker.substack.com/

You can also follow me on Instagram at:

https://www.instagram.com/seniorebiker/